Model Organisms in Plant Genetics

Edited by Ibrokhim Y. Abdurakhmonov

Published in London, United Kingdom

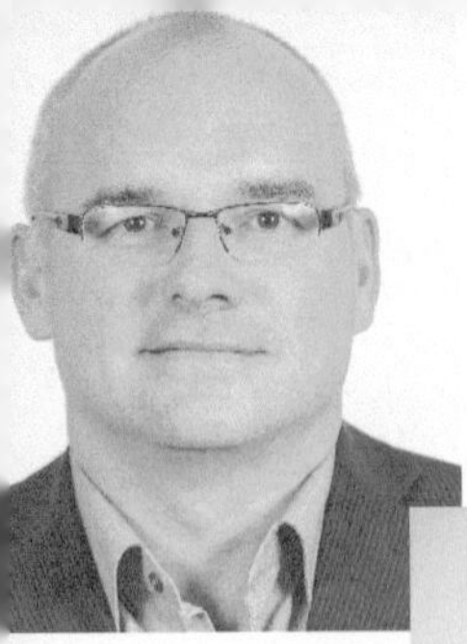
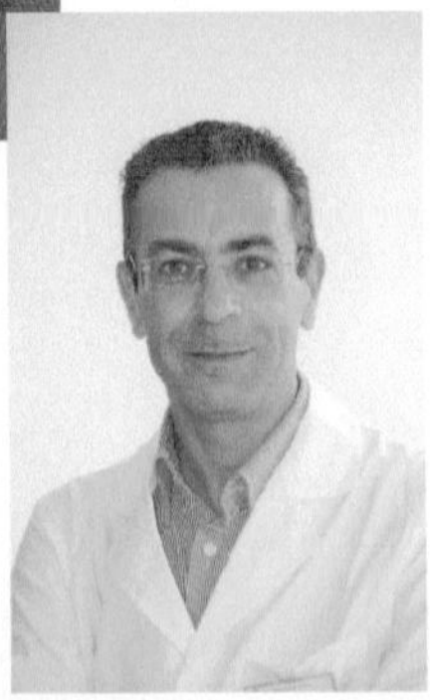
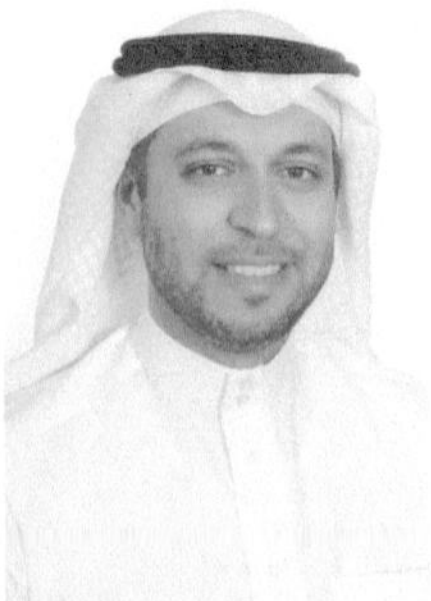
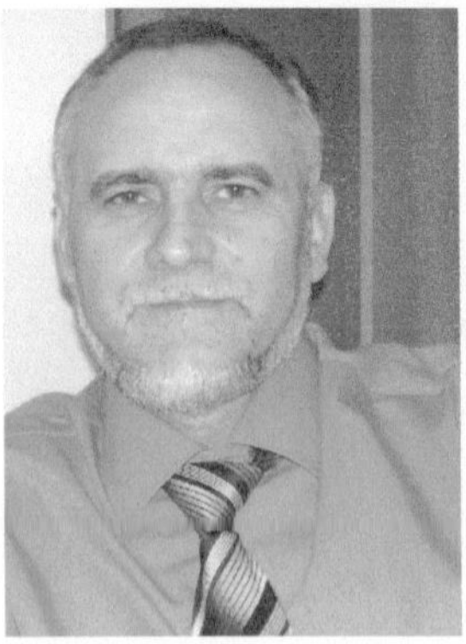
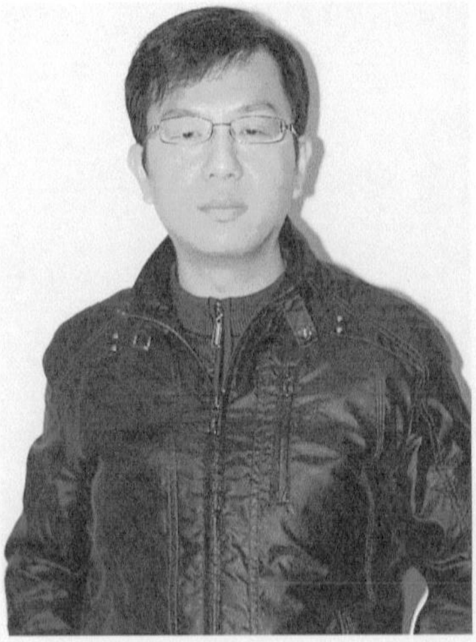
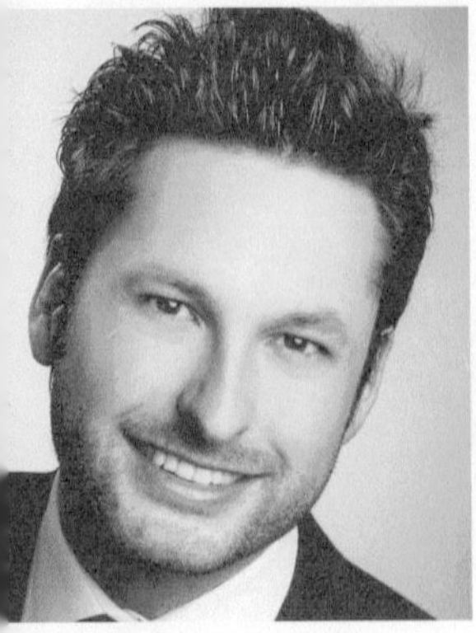
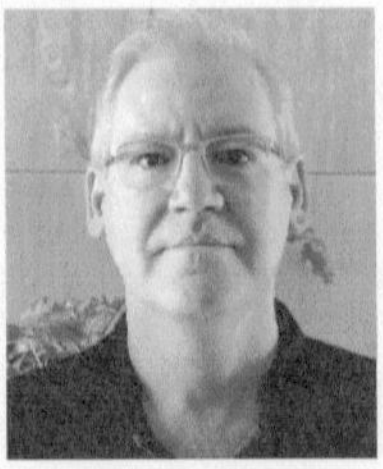

IntechOpen

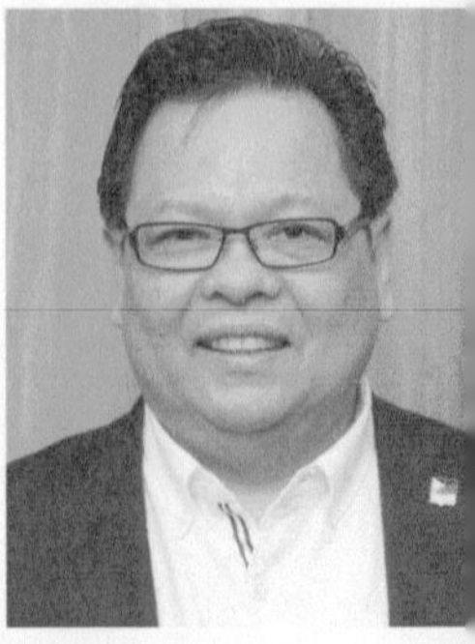
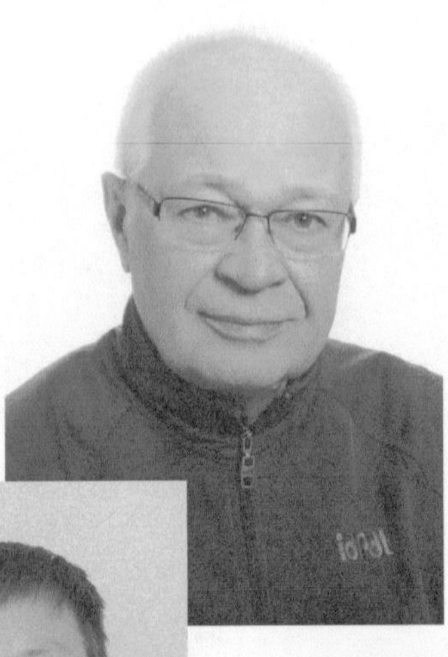
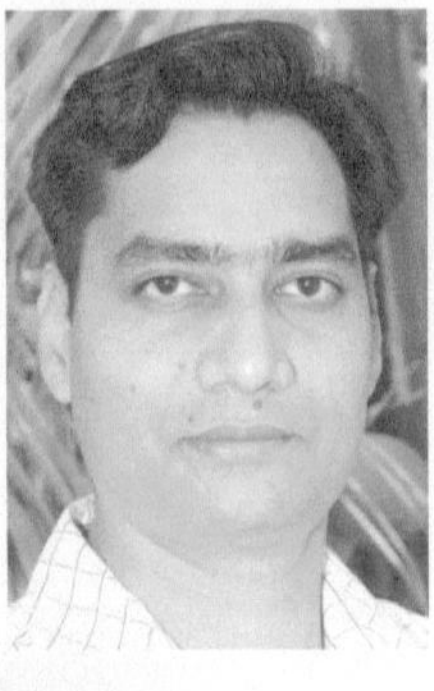
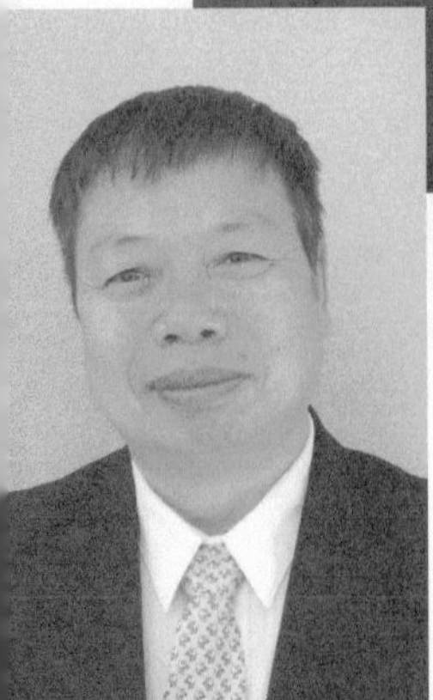
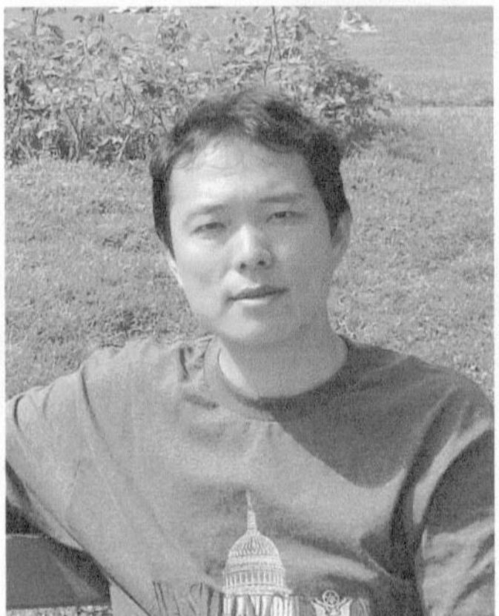
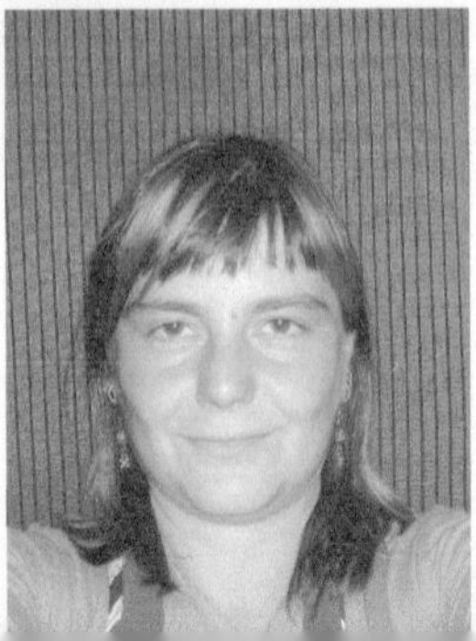

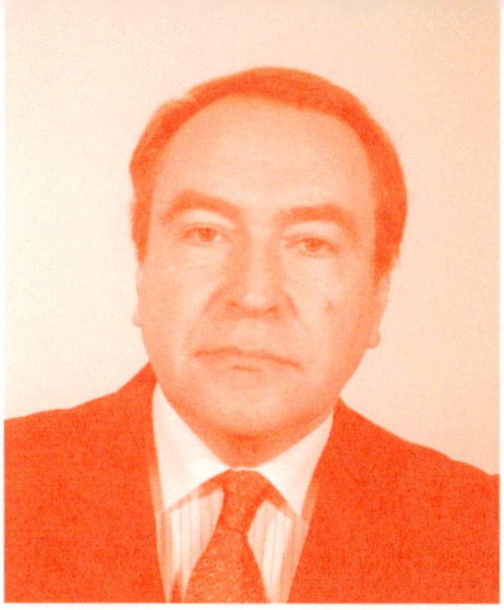

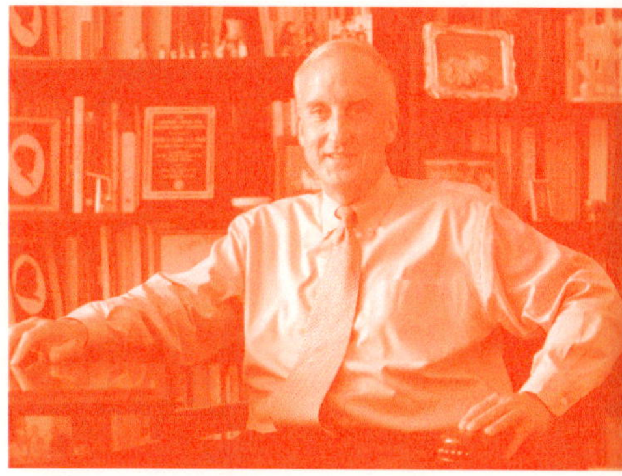

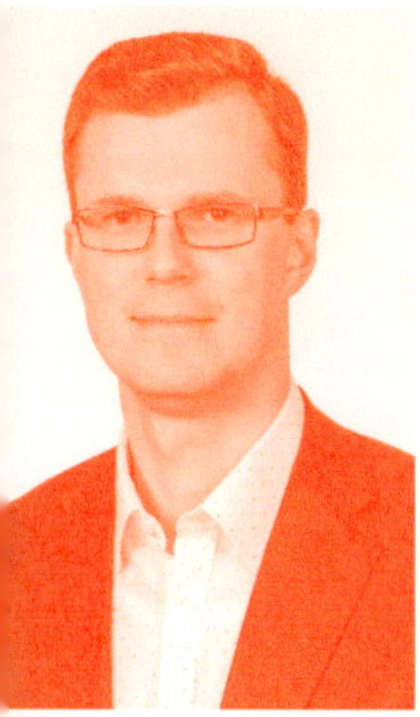

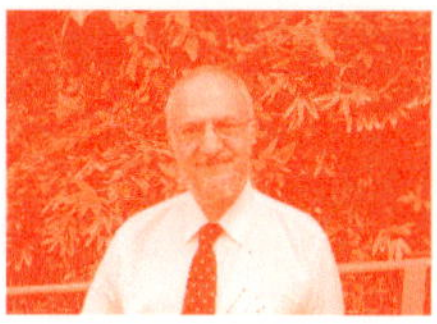

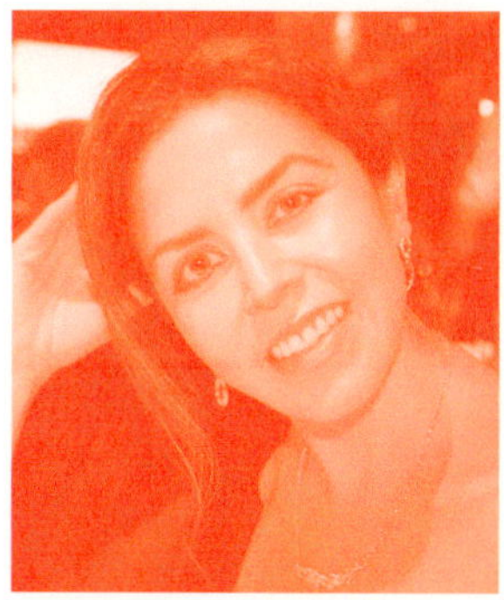

Supporting open minds since 2005

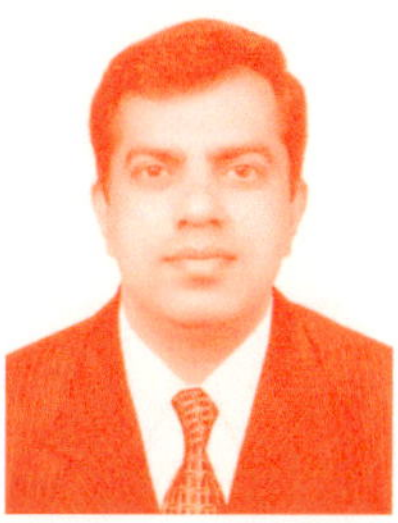

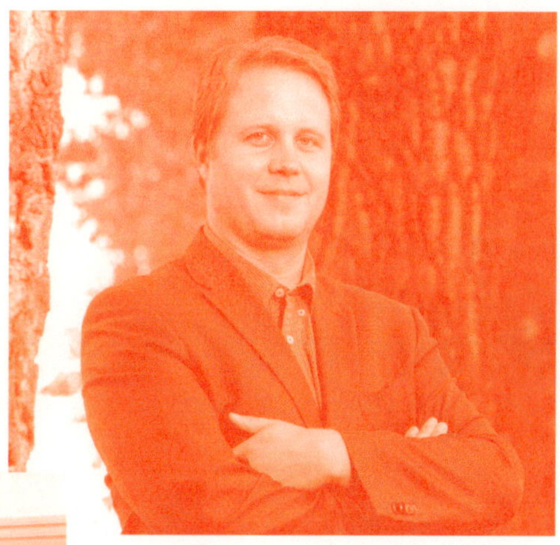

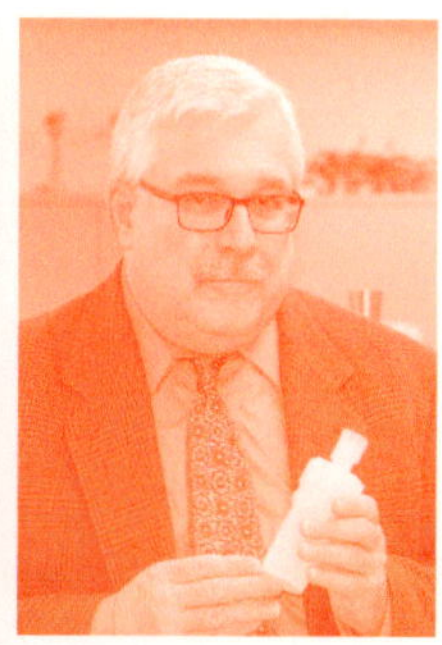

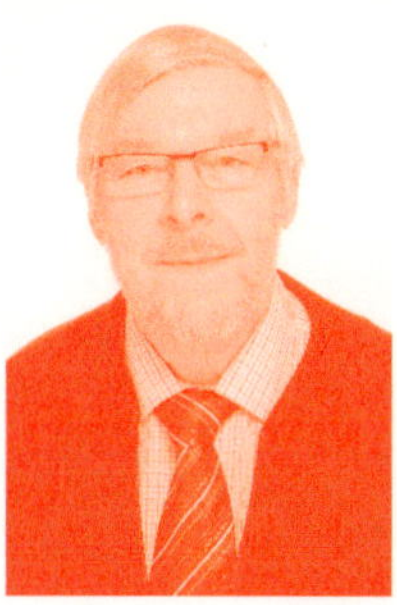

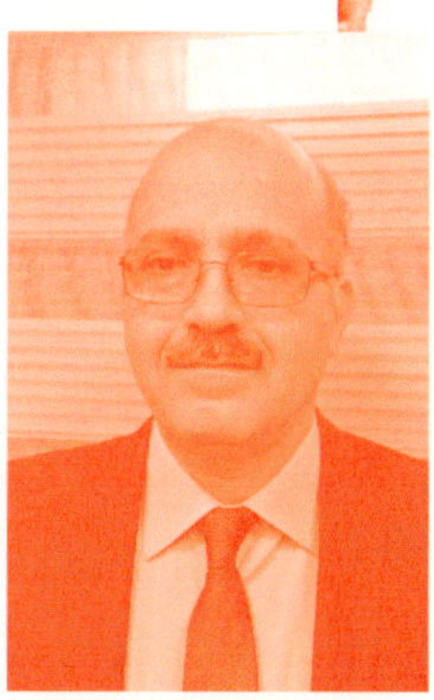

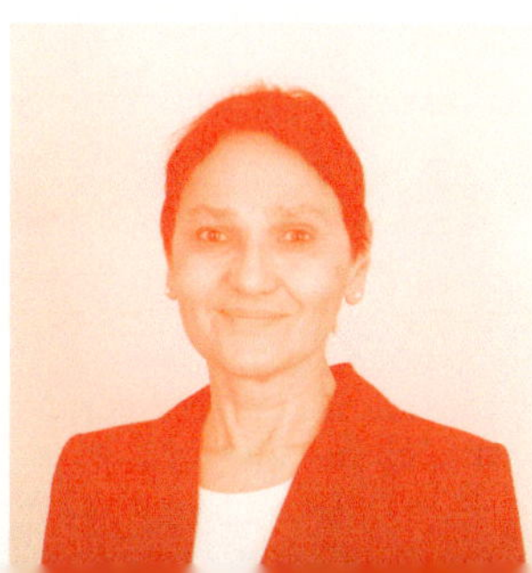

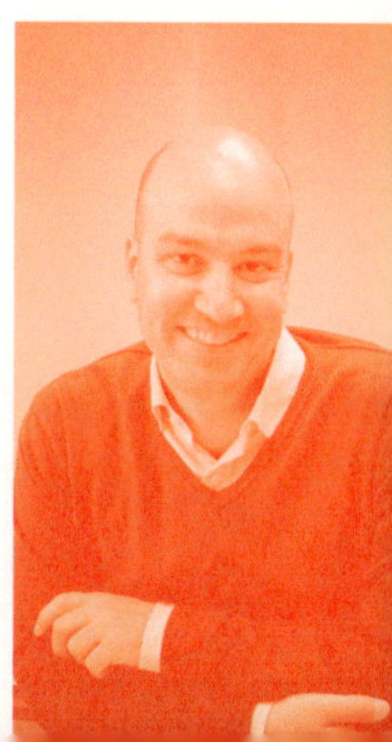

Model Organisms in Plant Genetics
http://dx.doi.org/10.5772/intechopen.94797
Edited by Ibrokhim Y. Abdurakhmonov

Contributors
Venera S. Kamburova, Ilkhom B. Salakhutdinov, Shukhrat E. Shermatov, Zabardast T. Buriev, Ibrokhim Y. Abdurakhmonov, Ayan Raichaudhuri, Madhabendra Mohon Kar, Fakhriddin N. Kushanov, Oybek A. Muhammadiyev, Nargiza M. Rakhimova, Ramziddin F. Umarov, Noilabonu N. Mamadaliyeva, Ozod S. Turaev, Guohao He, Sy M. Traore, Viola Willemsen, Jordi Floriach-Clark, Han Tang

First published in London, United Kingdom, 2022 by IntechOpen
IntechOpen is the global imprint of INTECHOPEN LIMITED, registered in England and Wales, registration number: 11086078, 5 Princes Gate Court, London, SW7 2QJ, United Kingdom
Printed in Croatia

British Library Cataloguing-in-Publication Data
A catalogue record for this book is available from the British Library

Additional hard and PDF copies can be obtained from orders@intechopen.com

Model Organisms in Plant Genetics
Edited by Ibrokhim Y. Abdurakhmonov
p. cm.
Print ISBN 978-1-83969-749-4
Online ISBN 978-1-83969-750-0
eBook (PDF) ISBN 978-1-83969-751-7

For EU product safety concerns:
IN TECH d.o.o., Prolaz Marije Krucifikse Kozulić 3, 51000 Rijeka, Croatia, info@intechopen.com or visit our website at intechopen.com.

Meet the editor

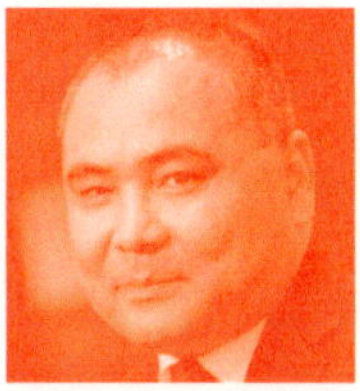

Ibrokhim Y. Abdurakhmonov received a BS in Biotechnology from the National University, California, in 1997, an MS in Plant Breeding from Texas A&M University in 2001, and a Ph.D. in Molecular Genetics, DSc in Genetics, and a full professorship in Molecular Genetics and Molecular Biotechnology from the Academy of Sciences of Uzbekistan in 2002, 2009, and 2011, respectively. He founded the Center of Genomics and Bioinformatics of Uzbekistan in 2012. He received the 2010 prize from The World Academy of Sciences (TWAS) and "ICAC Cotton Researcher of the Year 2013" for his outstanding contribution to cotton genomics and biotechnology. He was elected as a fellow to TWAS in 2014 and as a member of the Academy of Sciences of Uzbekistan in 2017. In the same year, he was appointed Minister of Innovative Development of Uzbekistan.

Contents

Preface

Model plants, among all other plant species, are very important for genetic studies to enhance understanding of plant life on our planet. Model plant species help researchers to study the genetics of key biological phenomena, processes, and characteristics. Plant models, as whole plants are grown from seed as well as tissue or cell culture, are used to experimentally investigate the consequences of natural mutations, adaptation of plants to harsh environments or changing climate, plant ecology and evolution, and polyploidization. Model organisms are particularly important when targeted plant species are difficult to study or when there is a lack of data. Because of the simplicity, suitability, and availability of research material for randomized and repeated experiments as well as the speed and precision of laboratory experiments, model plants are the key objects for plant science investigations.

Model plants with emerging new candidate species are widely used to simulate various morphological, physiological, and molecular processes in plants, allowing a more accurate understanding of the mechanisms underlying plant life. Furthermore, knowledge gained in studying model plants for key characteristics of interest can be generally translated to other plant species with the basic understanding that many key cellular and molecular processes are conserved and regulated by 'blueprint' genes inherited from a common ancestor.

Model Organisms in Plant Genetics discusses plant models for genetics and breeding research. Chapters describe characteristics of model plants such as *Arabidopsis*, moss, soybean, maize, and cotton, highlighting their advantages and limitations as well as their importance in studies of plant development, plant genome polyploidization, adaptive selection, evolution, and domestication, as well as in the improvement of industrially important traits. This book is a useful resource for students, life science researchers, and other interested readers.

I am thankful to the staff at IntechOpen, especially the Author Service Manager, Ms. Nera Butigan for her help throughout the editing process. I also thank all the chapter authors for their excellent contributions.

Ibrokhim Y. Abdurakhmonov
Center of Genomics and Bioinformatics,
Academy of Sciences of Uzbekistan,
Tashkent, Uzbekistan

Section 1

Introduction

Chapter 1

Introductory Chapter: Model Plants for Discovering the Key Biological Processes in Plant Research

Ibrokhim Y. Abdurakhmonov

1. Introduction

Model plants for genetic studies are very important among all other plant species living on our planet. Models, as the whole plant is grown from seed as well as tissue or cellular culture, help researchers to study the genetics of key biological phenomena, processes, and characteristics that are useful for understanding the consequences of natural mutations, adaptation of plants to the harsh environment or changing climate, plant ecology and evolution as well as polyploidization. Model organisms are particularly important and required when targeted plant species are very difficult to be easily studied or a needed research material is unavailable to be efficiently analyzed and data is generated; therefore, because of model plant simplicity, suitability, availability of research material for randomized and repeated experiments as well as speed and precision of laboratory experiments, model plants are "stand-in" [1] object for plant science investigations. Moreover, discovered biological and genetic functions of model plant species can be translated to the related plant taxa under the investigation due to orthologous and paralogous gene function and molecular cellular processes that can be extrapolated, explained, and varied by close or distant phylogenetic relationships.

2. Current status

One of the first model organisms for plant sciences was *Arabidopsis thaliana*, which was recognized as the universal model plant especially for all flowering eudicot plants due to short life cycle, ease of cultivation, relatively small genome size, and having a fully annotated genome sequence [1]. For the first time, studies on Arabidopsis as a model plant have begun to be carried out in the late 1970s. Currently, a search using the "plant models" keyword in the PubMed database has revealed more than 300 research publications on various model plants, including *A. thaliana* (**Figure 1**). A sharp increase in the number of publications on this topic has been observed since 2005, reaching a maximum in the last 5 years.

Since 2000, molecular genetic features of such biological processes as plant development, plant evolution, plant response to biotic and abiotic stresses, intracellular signaling, including hormonal signaling, were revealed using *A. thaliana* as a model plant [1]. In addition, *A. thaliana* is used as a model for studying the epigenetic regulation of metabolism [3]. In these studies, it was possible to establish the role

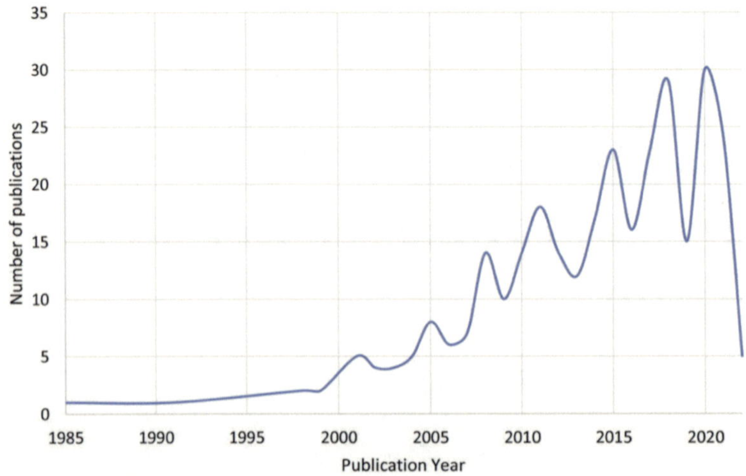

Figure 1.
Dynamics of "plant models" keyword-retrieved scientific publications. Source: PubMed [2].

of chromatin modification in the regulation of metabolism, as well as to identify metabolic pathways involving reactive oxygen species and nitric oxide (NO) in the modulation of chromatin activity under stress conditions [3].

However, the using of *A. thaliana* as a model plant is limited to Monocots and nonflowering plants due to strong differences in morphology, physiology, and genetics. Therefore, *A. thaliana* cannot be directly used to model studies on symbiotic interactions with soil microorganisms [1, 4]. All this prompted researchers to search for other model plants. So, at present, *Brachypodium distachyon* is used as a model for studying Monocots, mosses - *Physcomitrella patens*, legumes - *Medicago truncatula*, trees - *Populus trichocarpa* [1]. In addition, *Setaria viridis* is used to study C4 photosynthesis, the evolution of terrestrial plants – *Marchantia polymorpha* [1].

Additionally, currently, attention is being increasingly focused on the study of genomic multi-tissue metabolic models that allow to identify the metabolic interactions between tissues and organs [5]. Such models are developed for *Arabidopsis*, barley, soybean, and *Setaria*. Moreover, Arabidopsis-based models for metabolic pathways studies allow predicting the metabolic phenotype under genetic modifications, the course of metabolic reaction of plant tissues under changing environmental conditions [5]. Moreover, soybean-based multi-tissue models are used to study nutrient mobilization during seed germination. In addition, the model of using mesophyll and bundle sheath cells in *S. viridis* allows revealing the metabolic features of C4 photosynthesis [5].

Another interesting area of application of plant models is the study of allelopathy at the level of interaction both between individual plants and between organisms belonging to different kingdoms (plants, insects, fungi, and bacteria) [6]. Allelopathic plants (i.e., producing chemicals that inhibit the growth and development of other organisms) include wheat (*Triticum* sp.), rye (*Secale cereale*), corn (*Zea mays*), barley (*Hordeum vulgare*), rice (*Oryza sativa*), and sorghum (*Sorghum bicolor*). Of these plants, maize (Z. mays) is most often used as a model for studying allelopathy [6]. The use of allelopathic models made it possible to reveal the mechanism of stability and synergy of allelochemical substances, the dependence of their effect on biotic (soil bacteria) and abiotic (temperature, soil moisture, etc.) environmental factors.

Also, to study the synergistic or antagonistic interaction between organisms belonging to different kingdoms (plants, soil fungi, and bacteria), a system consisting of soybeans, rhizobacteria, and soil fungi are used as a model [7]. Such multi-component modeling made it possible to reveal the mechanisms of interaction between these organisms, including changes in the level of gene expression [7]. These results later can be used in agriculture to reduce the level of invasion by weeds and yield increase potential [6, 7].

Practical application in agriculture has received data on the features of the plants architecture and growth obtained using the so-called agent-based modeling [8–10]. These data made it possible to obtain plants with desired architecture and height and were used for such plants as kiwi (*Actinidia deliciosa*), apple (*Malus domestica*), avocado (*Persea americana* 'Hass'), peach (*Prunus persica*), grape (*Vitis vinifera*) [8–10]. *In silico* programs and platforms specially developed are used to process and optimize such numerical simulation models [11, 12].

3. Chapter topics

In this *Model Organisms in Plant Genetics* book, together with a group of international plant researchers, we successfully compiled the current status and view on the advance of plant models for genetics and breeding research. Chapter topics, presented herein, described advances on plant models characteristics of the mostly used plant Arabidopsis with its limitations and need for other types of model plants, views on how mosses are used for plant development studies. Several chapters describe how crops such as soybean, maize, and cotton can be a model for studying a group of industrially important traits such as oil production and plant genome polyploidization, adaptive selection, evolution, and domestication as well as crop improvement.

4. Conclusions

Thus, the last-five years' literature review, highlighted above, and new advances presented in chapters of this book, collectively highlight the importance and future key role of plant models for the development of plant sciences research, leading to novel discoveries. Model plants with emerging new candidate species will be widely used to simulate various morphological, physiological, and molecular processes in plants, allowing a more accurate understanding of the mechanisms explaining the plant ontogenesis.

Author details

Ibrokhim Y. Abdurakhmonov
Center of Genomics and Bioinformatics, Academy of Science of Republic of Uzbekistan, Tashkent, Uzbekistan

*Address all correspondence to: i.y.abdurakhmonov@gmail.com

References

[1] Cesarino I, Dello Ioio R, Kirschner GK, Ogden MS, Picard KL, Rast-Somssich MI, et al. Plant science's next top models. Annals of Botany. 2020;**126**(1):1-23. DOI: 10.1093/aob/mcaa063

[2] PubMed database [Internet]. 2021. Available from: http://www.ncbi.nlm.nih.gov/pubmed (Accessed: January 28, 2022).

[3] Lindermayr C, Rudolf EE, Durner J, Groth M. Interactions between metabolism and chromatin in plant models. Mol Metab. 2020;**38**:100951. DOI: 10.1016/j.molmet.2020.01.015

[4] Rensing SA. Why we need more non-seed plant models. The New Phytologist. 2017;**216**(2):355-360. DOI: 10.1111/nph.14464

[5] Shaw R, Cheung CYM. Multi-tissue to whole plant metabolic modelling. Cellular and Molecular Life Sciences. 2020;77(3):489-495. DOI: 10.1007/s00018-019-03384-y

[6] Schandry N, Becker C. Allelopathic Plants: Models for Studying Plant–Interkingdom Interactions. Trends in Plant Science. 2020;**25**(2):176-185. DOI: 10.1016/j.tplants.2019.11.004

[7] Afkhami ME, Almeida BK, Hernandez DJ, Kiesewetter KN, Revillini DP. Tripartite mutualisms as models for understanding plant–microbial interactions. Current Opinion in Plant Biology. 2020;**56**:28-36. DOI: 10.1016/j.pbi.2020.02.003

[8] Wang M, White N, Hanan J, He D, Wang E, Cribb B, et al. Parameter estimation for functional-structural plant models when data are scarce: Using multiple patterns for rejecting unsuitable parameter sets. Annals of Botany. 2020;**126**(4):559-570. DOI: 10.1093/aob/mcaa016

[9] Zhang B, DeAngelis DL. An overview of agent-based models in plant biology and ecology. Annals of Botany. 2020;**126**(4):539-557. DOI: 10.1093/aob/mcaa043

[10] Coussement JR, De Swaef T, Lootens P, Roldán-Ruiz I, Steppe K. Introducing turgor-driven growth dynamics into functional-structural plant models. Annals of Botany. 2018;**121**(5):849-861. DOI: 10.1093/aob/mcx144

[11] Picheny V, Casadebaig P, Trépos R, Faivre R, Da Silva D, Vincourt P, et al. Using numerical plant models and phenotypic correlation space to design achievable ideotypes. Plant, Cell & Environment. 2017;**40**(9):1926-1939. DOI: 10.1111/pce.13001

[12] Guo J, Xu S, Yan DM, Cheng Z, Jaeger M, Zhang X. Realistic Procedural Plant Modeling from Multiple View Images. IEEE Transactions on Visualization and Computer Graphics. 2020;**26**(2):1372-1384. DOI: 10.1109/TVCG.2018.2869784

Section 2

Widely Used Model Plants

Chapter 2

Overview of *Arabidopsis* as a Genetics Model System and Its Limitation, Leading to the Development of Emerging Plant Model Systems

Madhabendra Mohon Kar and Ayan Raichaudhuri

Abstract

Model plant systems make it easier to perform experiments with them. They help to understand and expand our knowledge about the genetic basis behind different plant process. Also, it is easier to design and perform genetic and genomic experiments using a model plant system. *A. thaliana* was initially chosen as the model plant system, and remains to this date, one of the most widely studied plant. With the advent of better molecular biology and sequencing tools and to understand the genetic basis for the unique processes in different plant species, there is emergence of several new model systems.

Keywords: Model plants, emerging model plants, genetic experiments, genomic studies, evolutionary model, legumes, crop plants, *Arabidopsis thaliana*, *Mimulus*, *Medicago truncatula*

1. Introduction

Model organisms are non-human species, which are usually less complex and easier to study to gain a broad understanding about different biological characteristics and phenomena [1]. The results obtained by studying the model organisms, are often used to understand the different biological characteristics and processes of the model of interest, which are usually more complex and difficult to study [1]. The term "model organism", came into use mostly in the 1990s with the advent of Human Genome Project [1]. The most widely, used model organisms that was recognized for biomedical research by National Institute of Health of USA, includes, thale cress (*A. thaliana*), mouse (*Mus musculus*), rat (*Rattus norvegicus*), zebrafish (*Danio rerio*), fruit fly (*Drosophila melanogaster*), nematode (*Caenorhabditis elegans*) and baker's yeast (*Saccharomyces cerevisiae*) [1].

Model organisms have several advantages that make it convenient to perform experiments with them [1, 2]. Some of those advantages include, being easier to grow and maintain in large numbers in labs, availability of different genetic strains, small genomic size, ease of performing genetic manipulations and ease of standardized isolation of genetic material and availability of thoroughly annotated genomes [1, 2]. Model organisms serve as useful tools for biological interventions, allowing easier experimental design and interpretation of genetic and genomic experiments. The understanding of the important role of genetics in plant research and the advent of powerful tools for molecular biology, pushed toward the need to focus on a single organism for performing detailed analysis [2, 3]. Use of a single model organism, also promoted interdisciplinary research, and helped in conserving resources required for research [2].

This chapter will provide a brief overview on *Arabidopsis* as a plant model system and its limitation, along with a brief overview of few emerging model plant system that are important in genetics research.

2. *Arabidopsis* as a plant model system

In the 1970s, the search for a model system in plant genetics, lead to interest in *Arabidopsis* research [2]. Several researchers and reviewers have shown interest and documented about the use of *A. thaliana* as a model organism, especially for genetic research [4–6]. *A. thaliana* has been the most used plant model systems for several decades [7]. This has allowed for extensive advances in the understanding of several biological process in plants, like, plant development, biotic and abiotic stress response, hormone biology and signaling [8]. Discoveries made as part of studying *Arabidopsis*, not only have been relevant to other plant species, but have also greatly enhanced the understanding of human biology [8–10].

Arabidopsis develop from a seed into mature plant, in a short period of time as six weeks [11]. Unlike many other plants, they can easily be grown indoors under feeble florescent lighting [11]. Also, the seed and seedlings of *Arabidopsis* is small, allowing the germination of the plant in an adequate number even on a single petri dish [11]. As the growth of this plant, requires no coculture of other species, it increases the possibility of controlling different variables and helps in maintaining aseptic growth conditions [11]. Thus, research using *Arabidopsis* is relatively convenient, fast, and cheap [2, 11]. The small genome size (~132 Mbp), along with the early availability of completed and annotated genome sequence of *Arabidopsis*, further made it central to genetic research [11, 12]. Also, the ability of the plant to undergo self-pollination and tolerate a high degree of homozygosity, makes it advantageous for research [2, 11].

Apart from genetics, *Arabidopsis* is also useful for answering questions about biochemistry, molecular biology, and physiology [13].

3. Limitations of using *Arabidopsis* as a model system

Moe than 400,000 species of gymnosperms, angiosperms, ferns, hornworts, lycophytes, mosses, liverworts, and algae, are classified as plants [7]. All of them, represents biodiversity in terms of their biochemistry, architecture, reproductive system and ecosystem among other characteristics [7]. *Arabidopsis* is a type of eudicot in the *Brassicaceae (Brassicales)* family, which along with monocots, are part of angiosperms (flowering plants) [7, 13]. It is a type of land plant. It is only one species of plant, that is only capable of growing in a certain limited set of environments [7]. So, to understand growth of different crop plants, and the evolutionary history of land plants, necessitates study of additional species [7].

Though many biological processes are common across various species of plant -- especially across flowering plants – several other processes are species or clade specific [13]. Some of those processes that varies widely across species, families, genera, and population are response to pathogens and plant secondary chemistry [13]. Also, some cereal crops that comprises as a major source of food, also varies morphologically, physiologically, and developmentally from *Arabidopsis* [13]. *Arabidopsis* does not have much symbiotic relation with soil microorganism as it does not associate with mutualistic arbuscular mycorrhizae [7, 11]. Also, it has an annual lifestyle, dicotyledonous way of development, and performs only C3 photosynthesis [7]. Also, not all genes that are expressed in other plants, are not represented in *Arabidopsis* [7]. Thus, having a single generic model cannot be used for understanding all aspects of plant biology.

4. Emerging plant models for studying genetics

4.1 *Brachypodium distachyon*

The tribe, Triticae, that includes crops like, wheat, barley, and rye, have large genomes, and are difficult to perform genetic studies on them [13]. *Brachypodium distachyon*, is closely related to wheat and barley (both belong to the tribe *Triticeae*, which are important crop plants, thus it was chosen as a model plant, to study cereal biology [13, 14]. It also has synteny with major small grains like, wheat, maize, millet, rice, and barley [15]. It is a small annual species, that belongs to the genus *Brachypodium* [13]. It is a C3 plant, that is distributed worldwide [15]. It has some characteristics that make it suitable to be used as a model system, to study genetics. The characteristics include, small genome size (~272 Mb), small size, ease of cultivation in lab and short lifecycle, ability to self-pollinate and ease of genetic crossings [13, 15]. The fully annotated reference genome sequence of *B. distachyon*, is publicly available [15]. Also, a large variety of tools are available to be used with this plant as a model system [13, 16–18]. They include availability of diverse collection of germplasm, microarrays, robust transformation protocol and several T-DNA insertion lines [13].

B. distachyon is an emerging model system that is useful for studying genetics of flowering plants [13]. This model system is particularly useful for understanding and expanding our knowledge about the biology of grasses, including that of small grains [15]. *B. distachyon* can serve as an essential system to study specific processes, like, endosperm development, cell wall biology, flowering control, and inflorescence development [13]. The plant is also useful for studying genetic basis for cold tolerance and genome organization, apart from the studying of loral development, vein patterning, the controls of the perennial versus annual habit [13]. There are several works, that describe the development of this plant as a model system [19–22].

4.2 *Medicago truncatula*

Though legumes are an important source of food apart from playing a major role in nitrogen fixation, most cultivated legumes are poor model systems for genomic research [23]. *Arabidopsis*, the most used plant model system cannot be used to proper understand many of the features uniquely seen in legumes [23, 24]. To study the rhizome legume symbiosis, Barker et al., suggested using *Medicago truncatula* as a model plant system [25, 26]. The plant possesses several features, that make it an ideal candidate for studying legume biology and genetics [24]. Some of them are, it's small genome size (~375 Mbp), that is sequenced and fully annotated, diploid genome, autogamous fertilization, relatively short generation time (around 4 months), rapid reproductive cycle, availability of large number of cultivars and presence of a well characterized nitrogen-fixing symbiont, *Sinorhizobium meliloti*

[24, 25, 27–30]. Also, the genus *Medicago* belongs to the phylum Galegoid [31]. So, it is related to several crop legumes like pea, chickpea, faba bean, lentil, chickpea, and clover [31]. Also, as members of this phylum have a similar genetic organization and high level of nucleotide sequence conservation, there is potential for easy transfer of genome sequence between the member species [24].

Several bioinformatics resources are available for *Medicago* like Medicago Gbrowser, LegumeGRN legumeIP, and Legoo [25]. Also, in addition to transcriptomics tools, several libraries for metabolic studies and reference maps for proteomic studies are available for *Medicago truncatula* [25, 32–34]. The capacity of the plant to be transformed efficiently and the generation of different mutants, have enhanced the ability to perform function genetic studies on *Medicago truncatula* [25]. *M. truncatula*, which is a legume related to alfalfa, has emerged as an important model plant, for studying and understanding the molecular biology and genetics of various processes involved in mycorrhizal, rhizobial, and pathogenic plant-microbe interactions [24]. To understand the biological processes like symbiotic nitrogen fixation (involving root nodule formation), the seed development, and the abiotic stress tolerance, genetic studies using *M. truncatula* is ideal [25].

4.3 *Mimulus*

Mimulus (monkeyflower) genus is important not only as a classic ecological and evolutionary model system but is also important for studying the developmental genetics and evolutionary development of certain important plant traits, that are not found in common model plant system like *Arabidopsis* [35]. Genetic studies with *Mimulus* could help to answer a large range of evolutionary and ecological questions [36].

The species within the genus *Mimulus* has become important for understanding the genetics of mating system evolution, speciation, inbreeding depression, ecological adaptations, cytological patterns of evolution and speciation [36–42]. This system is also phylogenetically attractive for broad comparative genomics research across the plant kingdom [36]. Species within mimulus has several attributes that facilitate genetic experimentation [36]. Such, attributes include the ability of several species within the genus being self-compatible, many can be clonally propagated using cuttings and short generation time under experimental conditions [36]. The *M. lewisii* complex, is currently best developed to be used as a model system among all the other *Mimulus* species – which includes the bumblebee-pollinated *M. lewisii*, hummingbird pollinated *M. cardinalis* and *M. verbenaceus*, and self-pollinated *M. parishii* -- for studying developmental genetics and evolutionary development [35]. This is owing to their characteristics like, these species being genetically similar enough to allow manual cross pollination to produce fertile offspring. They are also, uniquely suitable for genetic analysis as they have high fecundity (up to 1000 seeds per flower), short generation time (2.5–3 months), and small genome size (*c*. 500 Mb) [35].

The *M. lewisii* complex is used as a model system, to enhance our understanding in several research areas like, that of, regulation of carotenoid pigmentation, formation of periodic pigmentation patterns, developmental genetics of corolla tube formation and elaboration and molecular basis of floral trait variation underlying pollinator shift [35].

5. Future perspective

Model plant systems are important for studying and understanding the molecular biology and genetics of various plant processes. The definition of model systems and the list of model systems are changing with the increase in our understanding about plant processes and the advent of newer technologies to study plants [7]. The limitations of classical genetic manipulation that catapulted *A. thaliana* as a model plant system, are being addressed with the development of rapid high throughput genome sequencing and targeted gene editing using tools like TALENs, ZINC-FINGER nucleases, and CRISPR/Cas9 [7, 25]. This enables, a wider variety of plant species to be studied, and that helps to gain insights into unique and varied biological processes. The extensive use of emerging sequencing technologies, along with genomics and systems biology approaches will enhance understanding of the functional aspects of the gene pool of different plant species [25].

The technological advances, leading to the development of emerging model plants, will certainly help in providing more possibilities of choices to plant researchers. This will help in improving our understanding of the underlying genetics that influences the fundamental properties of plants and plant development. The increase in understanding, will increase our ability to genetically modify plants to better suit our needs.

Author details

Madhabendra Mohon Kar and Ayan Raichaudhuri*
Amity Institute of Biotechnology, Amity University, New Town, Kolkata, India

*Address all correspondence to: araichaudhuri@kol.amity.edu; ayan123@gmail.com

References

[1] Ankeny, R., & Leonelli, S. (2021). Model Organisms (Elements in the Philosophy of Biology). Cambridge: Cambridge University Press. doi:10.1017/9781108593014

[2] Koornneef, M. and Meinke, D. (2010), The development of Arabidopsis as a model plant. The Plant Journal, 61: 909-921. https://doi.org/10.1111/j.1365-313X.2009.04086.x

[3] Pruitt, R.E., Bowman, J.L. and Grossniklaus, U. (2003) Plant genetics: a decade of integration. Nat. Genet. 33, 294-304.

[4] Rédei, G.P. (1992) A heuristic glance at the past of Arabidopsis genetics. In Methods in Arabidopsis Research (Koncz, C., Chua, N.H. and Schell, J., eds). Singapore: World Scientific, pp. 1-15.

[5] Meinke, D.W., Cherry, J.M., Dean, C., Rounsley, S.D. and Koornneef, M. (1998) Arabidopsis thaliana: a model plant for genome analysis. Science, 282, 662-682.

[6] Pennisi, E. (2000) Arabidopsis comes of age. Science, 290, 32-35.

[7] Chang, C., Bowman, J. L., & Meyerowitz, E. M. (2016). Field Guide to Plant Model Systems. Cell, *167*(2), 325-339. https://doi.org/10.1016/J.CELL.2016.08.031

[8] Provart, N.J., Alonso, J., Assmann, S.M., Bergmann, D., Brady, S.M., Brkljacic, J., Browse, J., Chapple, C., Colot, V., Cutler, S., Dangl, J., Ehrhardt, D., Friesner, J.D., Frommer, W.B., Grotewold, E., Meyerowitz, E., Nemhauser, J., Nordborg, M., Pikaard, C., Shanklin, J., Somerville, C., Stitt, M., Torii, K.U., Waese, J., Wagner, D. and McCourt, P. (2016), 50 years of Arabidopsis research: highlights and future directions. New Phytol, 209: 921-944. https://doi.org/10.1111/nph.13687

[9] Piquerez, S. J. M., Harvey, S. E., Beynon, J. L., & Ntoukakis, V. (2014). Improving crop disease resistance: lessons from research on Arabidopsis and tomato. *Frontiers in Plant Science*, *0*(DEC), 671. https://doi.org/10.3389/FPLS.2014.00671

[10] Jones, A. M., Chory, J., Dangl, J. L., Estelle, M., Jacobsen, S. E., Meyerowitz, E. M., Nordborg, M., & Weigel, D. (2008). The Impact of Arabidopsis on Human Health: Diversifying Our Portfolio. Cell, *133*(6), 939-943. https://doi.org/10.1016/J.CELL.2008.05.040

[11] Andrew W Woodward, Bonnie Bartel, Biology in Bloom: A Primer on the *Arabidopsis thaliana* Model System, Genetics, Volume 208, Issue 4, 1 April 2018, Pages 1337-1349, https://doi.org/10.1534/genetics.118.300755

[12] Arabidopsis Genome Initiative, 2000

[13] Kellogg, E. A. (2015). Brachypodium distachyon as a Genetic Model System. *doi:10.1146/Annurev-Genet-112414-055135*, *49*, 1-20. https://doi.org/10.1146/ANNUREV-GENET-112414-055135

[14] Brkljacic J, Grotewold E, Scholl R, Mockler T, Garvin DF, et al. 2011. Brachypodium as a model for the grasses: today and the future. Plant Physiol. 157: 3-13

[15] Scholthof KBG, Irigoyen S, Catalan P, Mandadi KK. *Brachypodium*: A Monocot Grass Model Genus for Plant Biology. Plant Cell. 2018;30(8):1673-1694. doi:10.1105/tpc.18.00083

[16] Mur LA, Allainguillaume J, Catalán P, Hasterok R, Jenkins G, et al. 2011. Exploiting the Brachypodium tool

box in cereal and grass research. New Phytol. 191: 334-347

[17] Bevan MW, Garvin DF, Vogel JP. 2010. Brachypodium distachyon genomics for sustainable food and fuel production. Curr. Opin. Biotechnol. 21: 211-217

[18] Girin T, David LC, Chardin C, Sibout R, Krapp A, et al. 2014. Brachypodium: a promising hub between model species and cereals

[19] Vogel J.P. (2016). The rise of Brachypodium as a model system. In Genetics and Genomics of Brachypodium, Vogel J.P., ed (Switzerland: Springer;), pp. 1-7.

[20] Brutnell T.P., Bennetzen J.L., Vogel J.P. (2015). *Brachypodium distachyon* and *Setaria viridis*: Model genetic systems for the grasses. Annu. Rev. Plant Biol. **66**: 465-485.

[21] Kellogg E.A. (2015b). Brachypodium distachyon as a genetic model system. Annu. Rev. Genet.

[22] Lyons C.W., Scholthof K.-B.G. (2016). Brachypodium as an Arabidopsis for the grasses: Are we there yet? In Genetics and Genomics of Brachypodium, Vogel J.P., ed (Switzerland: Springer;), pp. 327-341.

[23] Benedito, V.A., Torres-Jerez, I., Murray, J.D., Andriankaja, A., Allen, S., Kakar, K., Wandrey, M., Verdier, J., Zuber, H., Ott, T., Moreau, S., Niebel, A., Frickey, T., Weiller, G., He, J., Dai, X., Zhao, P.X., Tang, Y. and Udvardi, M.K. (2008), A gene expression atlas of the model legume *Medicago truncatula*. The Plant Journal, 55: 504-513. doi:10.1111/j.1365-313X.2008.03519.x

[24] Thoquet, P., Ghérardi, M., Journet, EP. *et al.* The molecular genetic linkage map of the model legume *Medicago truncatula*: an essential tool for comparative legume genomics and the isolation of agronomically important genes. BMC Plant Biol **2,** 1 (2002). doi:10.1186/1471-2229-2-1

[25] Kang, Y., Li, M., Sinharoy, S., & Verdier, J. (2016). A Snapshot of Functional Genetic Studies in Medicago truncatula. *Frontiers in Plant Science*, *0*(AUG2016), 1175. doi:10.3389/FPLS.2016.01175

[26] Boisson-Dernier, A., Chabaud, M., Garcia, F., Bécard, G., Rosenberg, C., and Barker, D. G. (2001). *Agrobacterium rhizogenes*-transformed roots of *Medicago truncatula* for the study of nitrogen-fixing and endomycorrhizal symbiotic associations. Mol. Plant Microbe Interact. 14, 695-700. doi:10.1094/MPMI.2001.14.6.695

[27] Young, N. D., Debellé, F., Oldroyd, G. E. D., Geurts, R., Cannon, S. B., Udvardi, M. K., et al. (2011). The Medicago genome provides insight into the evolution of rhizobial symbioses. Nature 480, 520-524. doi:10.1038/nature10625

[28] Prosperi JM, Auricht G, Génier G, Johnson R: Medics (*Medicago* L.). In: Plant Genetic Resources of Legume in the Mediterranean (eds N. Maxted and S.J. Bennett), Kluwer Academic Publishers. 2001, 99-114.

[29] Sagan M, Morandi D, Tarenghi E, Duc G: Selection of nodulation and mycorhizal mutants in the model plant *Medicago truncatula* Gaertn after gamma rays mutagenesis. Plant Science. 1995, 111: 63-71. 10.1016/0168-9452(95)04229-N.

[30] Liu H, Trieu AT, Blaylock LA, Harrison MJ: Cloning and characterization of two phosphate transporters from *Medicago truncatula* roots: regulation in response to phosphate and to colonization by arbuscular mycorrhizal (AM) fungi. Mol Plant Microbe Interact. 1998, 11: 14-22.

[31] Doyle JJ, Doyle JL, Ballenger JA, Palmer JD: The distribution and phylogenetic significance of a 50 kb chloroplast DNA inversion in the flowering plant family Leguminosae. Mol Phylogenet Evol. 1996, 5: 429-438. 10.1006/mpev.1996.0038.

[32] Broeckling, C. D., Huhman, D. V., Farag, M. A., Smith, J. T., May, G. D., Mendes, P., et al. (2004). Metabolic profiling of *Medicago truncatula* cell cultures reveals the effects of biotic and abiotic elicitors on metabolism. J. Exp. Bot. 56, 323-336. doi: 10.1093/jxb/eri058

[33] Watson, B. S., Asirvatham, V. S., Wang, L., and Sumner, L. W. (2003). Mapping the proteome of barrel medic (*Medicago truncatula*). Plant Physiol. 131, 1104-1123. doi:10.1104/pp.102.019034

[34] Gallardo, K., Le Signor, C., Vandekerckhove, J., Thompson, R. D., and Burstin, J. (2003). Proteomics of *Medicago truncatula* seed development establishes the time frame of diverse metabolic processes related to reserve accumulation. Plant Physiol. 133, 664-682. doi:10.1104/pp.103.025254

[35] Yuan, Y.-W. (2019), Monkeyflowers (*Mimulus*): new model for plant developmental genetics and evo-devo. New Phytol, 222: 694-700. doi:10.1111/nph.15560

[36] Wu, C., Lowry, D., Cooley, A. *et al.* *Mimulus* is an emerging model system for the integration of ecological and genomic studies. Heredity **100,** 220-230 (2008). doi:10.1038/sj.hdy.6801018

[37] Sweigart AL, Fishman L, Willis JH (2006). A simple genetic incompatibility causes hybrid male sterility in *Mimulus*. Genetics **172**: 2465-2479.

[38] Bradshaw HD, Otto KG, Frewen BE, McKay JK, Schemske DW (1998). Quantitative trait loci affecting differences in floral morphology between two species of monkeyflower (*Mimulus*). Genetics **149**: 367-382.

[39] Dudash MR, Carr DE (1998). Genetics underlying inbreeding depression in *Mimulus* with contrasting mating systems. Nature **393**: 682-684.

[40] Fishman L, Kelly AJ, Willis JH (2002). Minor quantitative trait loci underlie floral traits associated with mating system divergence in *Mimulus*. Evolution **56**: 2138-2155.

[41] Angert AL, Schemske DW (2005). The evolution of species' distributions: reciprocal transplants across the elevation ranges of *Mimulus cardinalis* and *M. lewisii*. Evolution **59**: 1671-1684.

[42] Beardsley PM, Schoenig SE, Whittall JB, Olmstead RG (2004). Patterns of evolution in Western North American *Mimulus* (Phrymaceae). Am J Bot **91**: 474

Chapter 3

Mosses: Accessible Systems for Plant Development Studies

Jordi Floriach-Clark, Han Tang and Viola Willemsen

Abstract

Mosses are a cosmopolitan group of land plants, sister to vascular plants, with a high potential for molecular and cell biological research. The species *Physcomitrium patens* has helped gaining better understanding of the biological processes of the plant cell, and it has become a central system to understand water-to-land plant transition through 2D-to-3D growth transition, regulation of asymmetric cell division, shoot apical cell establishment and maintenance, phyllotaxis and regeneration. *P. patens* was the first fully sequenced moss in 2008, with the latest annotated release in 2018. It has been shown that many gene functions and networks are conserved in mosses when compared to angiosperms. Importantly, this model organism has a simplified and accessible body structure that facilitates close tracking in time and space with the support of live cell imaging set-ups and multiple reporter lines. This has become possible thanks to its fully established molecular toolkit, with highly efficient PEG-assisted, CRISPR/Cas9 and RNAi transformation and silencing protocols, among others. Here we provide examples on how mosses exhibit advantages over vascular plants to study several processes and their future potential to answer some other outstanding questions in plant cell biology.

Keywords: bryophyte, moss, model organism, plant development, regeneration, cell polarity, reprogramming, asymmetric division, stem cell, water-to-land, 2D-to-3D

1. Introduction

1.1 Mosses in context

Mosses are plants that belong to the Bryophytes, a cosmopolitan sister group of vascular plants with the last common ancestor between 400 and 500 million years ago [1, 2]. As a mostly avascular lineage, Bryophytes, that include mosses, liverworts and hornworts, thrive in mostly moist niches near the surface and stay compact (<10 cm), with some neovascularised exceptions that grow up to 65 cm [3–5]. Their cosmopolitan distribution in a variety of biotopes including moist and arid environments, can be explained by unique adaptations like drought, freezing and salinity tolerance [4, 6, 7]. Mosses' life cycle is dominantly gametophytic (the photosynthetic and growing phase is haploid), and the size and architecture of their organs is smaller and simpler than that of vascular plants, with leaf-like structures (phyllids) and sexual organs (antheridia and archegonia) of often only one cell of thickness, stem-like structures of circa ten cells and spore-bearing containers (sporangia) of single-cell spores [4, 8–10].

This miniaturised body renders mosses accessible systems for the study and dissection of cell and molecular aspects of plant biology that require close monitoring in time and space [11]. Such studies greatly benefit of the accessibility to single cells in a multicellular context. For instance, asymmetric and directional cell divisions are key life developmental tools to build an organism, but we lack understanding on how these processes are exactly controlled and regulated [12]. Importantly, these developmental drivers are shared between mosses and vascular plants, and to some extent with animals, and associated gene functions seem to be highly conserved despite the long period of independent evolution [13].

In the last two decades, mosses have gained high interest in plant research, with *Physcomitrium patens* (Hedw.) Mitten becoming a central model system. *P. patens* organelle genomes were sequenced in 2003 (plastids) and 2007 (mitochondria) and nuclear genome in 2008, with the latest revision in 2018. In addition to this, a myriad of genetic tools has emerged that allow close study of all processes of this moss as a representative of this lineage of the Bryophytes.

Hereby, we present how mosses, thanks to their simplified body plan and genetic networks in development, and with special focus in *P. patens*, can become cornerstone model organisms to study several developmental processes that determine plant architecture of most land plants [11]. We selected a number of outstanding developmental processes that pose central research questions in developmental biology of plants and that started to be investigated in mosses in the last years. These processes are introduced in a bottom-up approach, with special attention to their molecular and cellular basis, going from the early stages to the final plant organisation, chronologically. The essential and most used tools available to investigate these aspects of mosses are briefly described to facilitate the initiation into this model system. Finally, we show how the moss revolution has recently started with the rise in moss genomes sequenced and increase in moss research with additional species and questions beyond *P. patens*.

1.2 Moss morphology and life cycle

As most land plants, mosses have alternating generations between the haploid gametophyte and diploid sporophytes. However, unlike vascular plants, mosses spend most of their life cycle in the gametophytic stage, in which most of the organism asexual development, including photosynthesis and growth, occurs. The sexual organs eventually develop at this stage to give rise to the embryo after fertilisation, that produces the sporophyte over the gametophyte. This fruiting stage is diploid until haploidisation in spore formation takes place [11, 14].

Starting from a spore, the first developmental stage of the moss is the chloronema, a chloroplast-rich and single cell-wide filamentous tissue that serves for initial colony expansion, early photosynthesis and nutrient absorption. The cells are slightly elongated (~80 μm long), and the intercellular cell walls are oriented perpendicular to the growth direction [15]. This filament eventually transitions to caulonema, a quick-growing filamentous cell type that have underdeveloped chloroplasts at early stage, with longer and narrower cells (~250–300 μm long) that grow twice as fast, and with oblique intercellular cell walls [15–17]. This tissue has exploratory purposes and is favoured in stressful, light-poor, and nutrient-poor conditions, possibly with the aim of finding more suitable conditions [18, 19]. Caulonema can transition again to (secondary) chloronema [17]. The filamentous tissues are collectively referred to as protonemata and can laterally grow and divide to branch as new filaments. The protonemata grow in a mat-like fashion that shapes the two-dimensional (2D) developmental stage of mosses where the growth is confined in a plane of few millimetres of thickness.

Sometimes, the lateral cell outgrowth (the cell initial) gives rise to a bud cell instead of a branch cell, which is the beginning of gametophore development and the transition to three-dimensional (3D) growth [20]. The identity of the cell initial can be predicted by the division plane angle, implying that identity is determined before division (**Figure 1**). Currently, the list of known genes involved in the path selection and division plane orientation is growing, but the early determinants of bud formation and branching remain unknown [18, 21]. The bud grows by well-defined asymmetrical and oriented divisions to form the gametophore, the leafy shoot-like plantlet of mosses that ultimately bears gamete-producing organs.

The bud basal cell gives rise to a new type of filamentous tissue, the rhizoids, with pigmented, caulonema-like morphology. They function as anchorage to the ground to stabilise the up-growing gametophore and contribute to nutrient and water uptake, similar to roots and root hairs of seed plants, but with the tissue complexity of root hairs [22, 23]. The bud apical cells divide in precise directions to give rise to oriented phyllid initial cells with a particular phyllotactic pattern (i.e. lateral organ organisation around the shoot; e.g. spiral) to develop the gametophore.

The apical cells eventually arrest their proliferation, or terminally give rise to sexual organs (firstly antheridia, and later archegonia) under autumnal/spring conditions: short day (8 h), low light (20 $\mu mol/m^2/s$) and low temperature (15°C) [24, 25]. Despite the asynchronous development of male and female gametangia, this moss is self-fertilising, and thus tends to genetically self-isolate [26]. Flagella-driven spermatozoids (male gametes) move towards the archegonial venter in liquid water and fertilise the egg cell to give rise to a diploid zygote. The zygote will subsequently develop, via an embryonic stage with a new 2D-to-3D transition, into the sporophyte, that consists of the foot (the interface with the gametophyte) and a short stalk (seta) with a terminal capsule. In the capsule, meiosis gives rise to up to few thousands of haploid spores [8, 26].

The first documented ecotype, known as 'Gransden' (United Kingdom, 1962), has reduced rates of sporophyte formation, probably due to long asexual propagation in laboratories [27]. In many laboratory lineages, it has become self-sterile, rendering it unattractive for studies dependant on sexual reproduction. On the contrary, the more recently isolated ecotypes 'Villersexel' (France, 2003) and

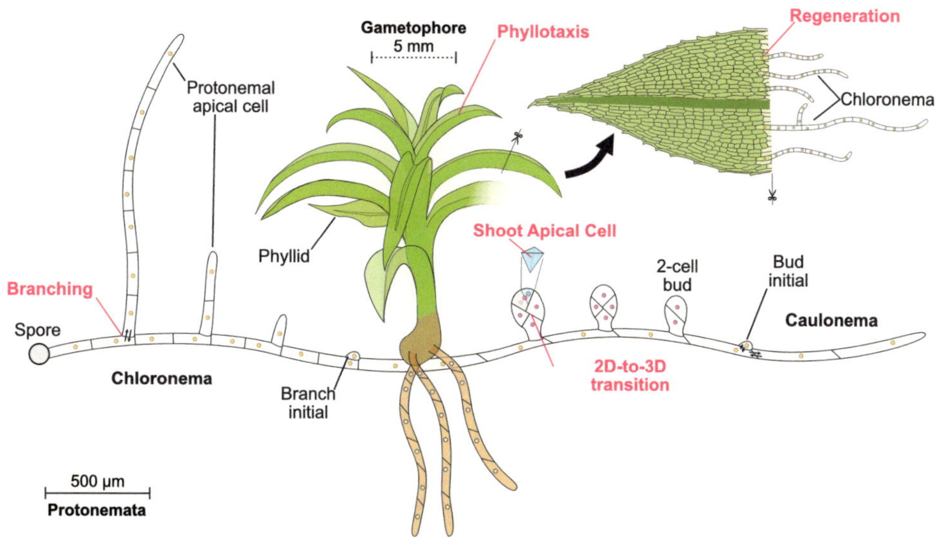

Figure 1.
Scheme of morphology and location of different developmental processes.

'Reute' (Germany, 2006) have 15 times more sporophytes (77% of total gametophores), indicating a high fertility rate [26]. Despite these differences, all ecotypes can be propagated asexually in identical conditions from any tissue thanks to the high regeneration rate of this moss, through which explants will redifferentiate into chloronema and initiate the life cycle from there [28, 29].

2. Outstanding developmental processes

Several essential developmental processes are shared between all land plants, including angiosperms and bryophytes. Strikingly, in mosses many shared processes take place with a simplified set of genes and sometimes in single cells. Therefore, the underlying genetic regulatory networks of development are easier to study. In this section, we highlight some of these processes and their unique ease of study in the moss *P. patens*.

2.1 The 2D-to-3D transition

The ability to structure organs in three dimensions (3D) was an essential feature for water-to-land transition. Many aquatic plants develop in a homogeneous environment, whereas land plants faced a highly distinct environment at ground surface level (a plane) and at the air/soil axis (perpendicular to this plane). This required land plants to develop specific tissues to efficiently grow in each dimension and cope with new challenges [20].

From a physiological perspective, the transition from 2D-to-3D growth in mosses consists in the development of complex structures such as the gametophore that grows out of the surface plane where protonema thrive, exhibiting negative gravitropism and positive phototropism [30–32]. The development of the gametophore relies on the ability of the moss to define different organisation in each dimension of space. The basal units from which this spatial assembly takes place are ultimately single cell primordia, from which organs emanate [33]. To this end, a cell must spatially sense intrinsic and extrinsic signals and transduce them to subcellular structures that pave the way to division plane positioning and subsequent asymmetric and oriented cell division. However, the molecular basis of spatial sensing and its transduction to organisation, action and maintenance of the division machinery has not been fully elucidated yet [12].

Cellularly, the 2D-to-3D transition in a moss occurs during bud formation (**Figure 1**). When a cell initial is formed in protonemata, in 5% of the cases it has a bud initial cell identity instead of a branch initial identity. Each bud initial swells and undergoes divisions oriented in all three axes of space [34]. This transition is supported and maintained by a different genetic and molecular machinery than that of protonemal development, and is the molecular basis of 3D growth. These proteins are specifically present from the first cell of the bud and onwards (e.g. DEK1, NOG1), and remains active in subsequent proliferating organs (e.g. shoot apical meristem, phyllids, gametangia) [13, 34–36]. In general, gradients or local clusters of proteins, peptides, nucleic acids, and hormones can be signals, sensors and/or actuators in developmental processes, and what is upstream of the cascade of 2D-to-3D transition remains a mystery. Some actors that are already on the radar include oscillations of auxin and cytokinin concentrations, ROP and SOSEKI proteins and CLE/CLV peptides-receptors, and they have been pinned down to different moments of the process and at different locations [12, 37, 38]. However, how do they coordinate their activity remains elusive and an active area of study.

In vascular plants, the 2D-to-3D transition occurs only once in their lifecycle, during embryogenesis, where orthologs of the essential moss 3D machinery genes are also expressed [34, 35]. This event is confined in the endosperm during embryogenesis and its observation in seed plants requires seed and ovule microdissection, which makes *in vivo* monitoring difficult [39]. Furthermore, knockouts of some of these genes are lethal in this early stage. On the contrary, *P. patens* exhibits both growth fashions (2D and 3D) simultaneously and frequent transition events (bud formation) during all its vegetative stage in each colony (months), and deletion or functional mutants are non-lethal due to the indefinite growth character of the remaining 2D tissues [34, 35].

These features provide a privileged seat for *in vivo* long-term tracking and subcellular study of molecular markers, gene expression and protein localization that allows to shed light to the necessary cellular events required establish 3D growth in single cells to build a full plant.

2.2 The shoot apical meristem/cell (SAM/SAC) assembly

The protagonist of 2D-to-3D growth transition is the formation of the shoot apical meristem (SAM), a region at the apical growth side responsible for the continuous formation of the aerial organs of the plant, including leaves and reproductive organs [40, 41]. The histology of the SAM in angiosperms describes a central zone with stem cells that self-renew, divide and radially differentiate into peripheral cells that determine organ initiation at specific locations (e.g. by placement and establishment of new leaf primordia) [42]. While angiosperms present multicellular stem cell centre SAMs during their sporophytic phase, bryophytes present an unicellular structure, the shoot apical cell (SAC), both in their gametophytic and sporophytic phase (**Figure 1**) [43]. Despite the differences, both SAM/SAC share a common organisation, with stem cell(s) at the centre, surrounded by regularly differentiating tissue [44].

The mechanisms that establish and maintain these pluripotent stem cell(s) in the SAM/SAC is unknown. It involves spatial sensing, cell-to-cell communication, and asymmetric and oriented cell divisions, which render mosses attractive systems for their accessibility. *De novo* establishment of SAC is especially easy to study in mosses because it occurs once per bud formation (hundreds of events per colony) and in sporophyte development after egg cell fertilisation (on top of ~77% of gametophores). These SAC establishment events consist of one relatively exposed cell, that is easy to monitor during several division rounds for weeks [16, 26]. Angiosperms present a SAM and numerous equivalent lateral meristems, sometimes big and manageable (e.g. cauliflower meristems), but in general their study requires dissection for visualisation and it consists of complex multicellular structures that complicate characterisation.

The developmental origin of the sporophytic SAC in *P. patens* is either a *de novo* SAC establishment after egg fertilisation or a gametophytic SAC redefinition [45, 46], and in any case the genetic and signalling basis and developmental mechanisms of its establishment seem conserved between angiosperms and bryophytes [22, 47].

The genetic make-up in both taxa has shown to rely on auxin response through AUXIN RESPONSE FACTORS (ARFs), cytokinin signalling by ARABIDOPSIS RESPONSE REGULATORS (ARRs), CHASE domain-containing histidine kinases (CHKs) and CYTOKININ OXIDASE/DEHYDROGENASE (CKX), local coordination through several transcription factors families like CLAVATAs (CLVs), CUP-SHAPED COTELYDONS (CUC), LATERAL ORGAN BOUNDARY (LOB) and signalling peptides like CLAVATA3/EMBRYO SURROUNDING REGIONRELATED (CLE) and chromatin modification by Polycomb Repressive Complex 1 and 2 (PRC1,2), among others [48]. Although many key factors have conserved roles in SAM formation and maintenance in seed plants and mosses, some important factors in angiosperms, like the key regulator of stem cell maintenance WUSCHEL, are not found in *P. patens*. These kind of differences can be insightful in defining the basic network to maintain *stemcellness*, tailoring a SAM and help understanding cell identity switch and organ formation [44].

2.3 Phyllotaxis from a cell

The most noticeable outcome of the shoot apical meristem/cell (SAM/SAC) activity is the organised and oriented initiation of leaf primordia along the stem, which leads to a unique geometric pattern of leaves and shoot branches named *phyllotaxis* [49]. In land plants, phyllotaxis may be defined by both genetic and environmental factors (light abundance, wavelength intensity ratio, etc.). For instance, leaf organisation can be adapted by shade avoidance syndrome [50]. However, only the genetic factors are shown to play a role in organ primordium location determination. A phyllotactic pattern is quantified by a fraction in which the denominator is the number of organs of the same type until the same orientation repeats (e.g. in *P. patens*, every fifth phyllid lies almost exactly below or above the first) and the numerator is the number of turns it takes (e.g. two turns in *P. patens*). This ratio (2/5) is then the fraction of a turn (e.g. 2/5 x 360°) or angle between two consecutive organs. When the angle between organs tends to the golden angle (137.5°, with fractions of turn derived from the Fibonacci sequence: 2/5, 3/8, 5/13, etc.), a spiral pattern emanates. Different angles can be observed in different species, like e.g. the 180° angle that gives rise to a distichous (or alternate) pattern or 120° for a tristichous pattern. Both Arabidopsis and *P. patens* follow a spiral pattern [43, 49, 51–53].

However, the pattern arises from essentially different SAMs/SACs: in angiosperms, phyllotaxis derives from a multicellular system with well-reported oscillating auxin peaks around the SAM growth axis, whereas *P. patens* effectively generates a pattern from a single apical cell (SAC). During the first division rounds in bud formation, the initial cell divides asymmetrically and gives rise to an inverted tetrahedral SAC with three lateral faces (**Figure 1**) [24, 54]. An oriented cell division of the SAC produces a new central SAC and a peripheral derivative cell, the merophyte, which develops into the future phyllid and a portion on the stem. The change of the stem cell division plane orientation in the SAC in each round results in a spiral phyllotactic pattern of the phyllids [55], which requires some unknown round-to-round cue to achieve rotation. Surprisingly, the rotation direction or chirality of the division orientations appears to be randomly determined, showing both clockwise (S) and counter clockwise (Z) patterns, yet there is high frequency of switch from one to the other (antidromy) in branches of gametophores of other moss species [56].

The limited understanding of the origin and underlying molecular mechanisms of this rotating pattern and derived phyllotactic pattern is largely confined to the sporophyte of the evolutionarily recent group of flowering plants (angiosperms). The available transcriptomic data of bud and tip cells and gametophores (or 3D shoots) may provide more insight in the transition from uniplanar to triplanar meristematic growth in moss [48].

Aligned with the phenotypic similarities of moss and angiosperm phyllotactic patterns, several factors known from Arabidopsis have also been found in mosses, including receptor signalling genes involved in shoot meristem size and patterning, hormone biosynthesis genes, transcription factors that control cell-specific mechanism of developmental pattering, chromatin remodelling complexes and cell cycle [48]. Many of these factors are essentially executive and likely controlled by some spatial sensing machinery. Comparing them with new contributors or absent members in the minimal regulatory network of mosses may help unravelling the fundamental elements that trigger the orientation-specification machinery that greatly impacts plant architecture in all land plants, including relevant crops.

2.4 Regeneration

Most described processes in this chapter require cell identity acquisition and maintenance. In certain circumstances (e.g. wounding), differentiated plant cells can reprogram to become new stem cells, divide and redifferentiate for organ *regeneration* [57, 58]. *P. patens* is an excellent system to investigate cell reprogramming and regeneration due to its fast and broadly occuring cell pluripotency [59].

In most tissue cultures of other plant species, exogenous hormones (e.g. auxin and cytokinin) are required to induce callus formation and plant regeneration [60]. However, in moss, cells are capable of regenerating from protoplasts or excised phyllids into new protonema filaments in the absence of exogenous hormones (**Figure 1**) [61]. This implies that the whole regeneration toolkit is present in mosses and can be endogenously activated on demand, which makes them different from other taxa (e.g. angiosperms) [62].

When a phyllid is excised, cells neighbouring the cutting edge can reprogram from somatic cells to protonemal stem cells, which can then start a new life cycle [14]. This regeneration process is easy to study in mosses for several reasons: firstly, cell identity conversion can be easily tracked with protonema stem cell reporters [29]; secondly, aside of the simplicity of *in vivo* observation (see section *Imaging*), the unistratose (i.e. single cell-layered) phyllid simplifies single-cellular extractions (e.g. laser ablation) for single cell *omics* and other high precision studies [63]. Interestingly, the result of the reprogramming cascade is timely visible 48 hours after cutting, which also allows large scale collection of excised tissue for time-course tracking of gene expression evolution during regeneration activation [64].

The mechanistic studies of the cell fate acquisition can benefit from this simple cell type conversion in comparison to other model systems used in cell reprogramming investigation (e.g. regenerative callus or Arabidopsis roots that consist of multiple cell types that possess different tissue identity) for its minimality and event frequency [65, 66]. In angiosperms, regeneration is often reduced to localised stem cell pools (e.g. the base of leaves), takes longer to establish, and it is multicellular and asynchronous at the explant level [58, 67].

Previous studies have taken advantage of the abovementioned features to investigate gene expression profile during phyllid cell reprogramming, which revealed that genes involved in stress, proteolysis, and hormone signalling pathways are induced from 6 to 24 h after cutting [64]. Some genes have been demonstrated to play essential roles in moss leaf reprogramming, including *Cyclin-dependent kinase A (CDKA),* found to link cell cycle reactivation and other cellular responses that promote cell outgrowth as a new protonema filament [29]. Similarly, the outgrowth of reprogrammed protonema cell requires *WUSCHEL-related homeobOX 13-Like (WOX13L)* genes and *Cold-Shock domain Protein 1 (PpCSP1)*, induced in the cells facing the cutting edge within 24 h [68, 69]. Finally, an AP2/ERF transcription factor *STEMIN1 (STEM CELL-INDUCING FACTOR 1)* was discovered to induce cell reprogramming in moss leaves without excision or wounding [70]. These studies have identified new pieces in the puzzle of cellular reprogramming, and future studies will aim to unravel mechanisms behind the cell identity conversion and reprogramming.

One interesting feature of moss regeneration is inhibition of neighbouring cells. The necessary cell–cell (apoplastic e.g. Ca^{2+}-mediated) or cell-to-cell (plasmodesmata-mediated) communication makes regeneration an attractive developmental process to study this cell crosstalk [71–73]. The phytohormone ABA is a key responsible of the dynamic regulation of the permeability of plasmodesmata in response to changing environments, such as wounding. Control in plasmodesmata pore size can influence the signalling molecules that can pass through or can be blocked in particular cells, which can have a direct effect in development of the processes mentioned until now [74, 75].

2.5 Hormone regulation

The signalling pathways and functions of plant hormones are substantially conserved in *P. patens*. Given the differences in physiological structures and relative evolutionary positions between angiosperms and bryophytes, mechanistic studies of hormone regulation in mosses can bring new insights in the hormone regulatory networks of all plants that resolve current questions.

Three plant hormones—auxin, cytokinin and strigolactone—have shown to regulate shoot branching patterns (phyllotaxis) and activation in angiosperms. Auxin moves down the main shoot of angiosperms to inhibit branch development, while cytokinin promotes branching. In addition to branching, auxin is the key molecule in the control of plant growth and development, and promotes organ differentiation [76, 77]. Exogenous application of auxin or its inhibitors results in irregular cell shapes and inhibit lateral organ formation, for instance in shoot apical meristem (SAM) maintenance. The understanding of hormone regulation and signalling in angiosperms progresses slowly due to tissue and gene network complexity. In *P. patens* interfering with auxin transport via the auxin efflux protein PIN-FORMED (PINs) knock-outs reveals the same effects on SACs as that have been observed in Arabidopsis SAMs. Also, the interaction between core components in auxin signalling and their response to auxin in *P. patens* is also conserved when compared to Arabidopsis [78–80]. Furthermore, exogenous application of auxin leads to termination of gametophore and differentiation into rhizoids, as it happens with shoots and roots in Arabidopsis [81]. In protonema cells, PIN-mediated auxin transport is essential for the chloronema-to-caulonema transition. When PINs are overexpressed, tip auxin levels deplete, which results in cell fate transition inhibition, while the PIN knock-out mutants show a faster transition from chloronema to caulonema [82]. Despite of these similarities, it has been shown that mosses may not weave their architecture with PIN-based transport as angiosperms do. On the contrary, they require bi-directional auxin transport to generate the observed patterns of shoot branching, as was confirmed by modelling and empirical evidence [83]. It derives that plasmodesmata-based transport may play a key role, which renders cell-to-cell communication essential in plant architecture definition and has not been reported in angiosperms [83].

Cytokinins and strigolactones also influence plant architecture, both in angiosperms and mosses. The levels of cytokinin are high and precisely distributed in the central stem cell region of SAM in angiosperms to maintain stemcellness [84]. In the root apical meristem, auxin and cytokinin act antagonistically in meristem size control, but its levels, distribution and interaction in *P. patens* single apical cell environment are unknown. Despite that, both hormones are present in this moss and are likely to play a role. The application of high concentrations of cytokinin in culture causes ectopic shoot formation and inhibition of leaf formation [83, 85]. Also, in gametophore development, cytokinin inhibits rhizoid formation by opposing auxin, like in roots of Arabidopsis. As expected by this homologous functionality, the mutants that stimulate cytokinin degradation lead to a strong increase of rhizoids in both number and length [86]. The last mentioned hormone, strigolactone, is reported to inhibit shoot branching in angiosperms and its localisation is restricted to the base of shoots. The same compound is able to stimulate the pattern of shoot branching in *P. patens*. In filamentous tissues, strigolactone is produced to inhibit chloronema branching and to regulate the colony extension [15, 87].

As shown, many processes that define plant architecture are regulated in similar ways both in angiosperms and mosses. However, mosses offer a reduced gene network and regulation complexity that facilitates the analysis of hormone functions in the related developmental processes. Furthermore, subcellular and tissue-level transport and distribution of hormones can be best visualised in their simple plant bodies. In such plant models, new hormone functions will prove to be easier to study and translate to agronomically relevant plants.

3. Protocols and tools

Many valuable online resources with information on protocols, stocks, tools and genetic information have been exhaustively compiled elsewhere [11]. Hereby, we provide some additional information and summary of the essentials of research in *P. patens*.

3.1 Imaging

3.1.1 Accessibility

The small size and simple architecture of moss organs allows detailed microscopic visualisation easy to accomplish in almost all tissues. The strings of cells in protonema and their branching is trivial to closely visualise, and the transition to gametophores can be well tracked until the stem-like centre becomes slightly thicker than a dozen of cells and grows out of the plane. From it, the leaf-like structures (phyllids) have only one cell of thickness except in the midrib and can be tore apart for up-close visualisation. The terminal sexual organs (antheridia and archegonia) have a 3D structure that is easy to fully dissect or directly visualise due to their monolayered sack structures. The subsequently developed spore-bearing containers (sporangia) are full of single-cell spores [4].

This miniaturised body renders mosses accessible systems for the study and dissection of cell and molecular biology that require close monitoring in time and space. Such studies greatly benefit of accessibility to single cells in their context for observation of subcellular responses *in vivo,* e.g. protein localization, cytoskeleton rearrangement, and cell divisions along the developmental progress in a better resolution than most other multicellular plant tissues.

3.1.2 Reporter or marker lines

In *P. patens*, fluorescent marker lines that label different organelles (e.g. ER, chloroplasts, mitochondria, peroxisomes, Golgi apparatus, vacuoles, and nucleus) are available. In addition, given the predictable division patterns of the protonema tip cells, *P. patens* has been extensively used to investigate mitosis. Therefore, marker lines containing fluorescently labelled proteins such as several microtubule-associated proteins relevant to cell divisions were generated for mitosis imaging. Other published reporter lines show the concentration of the hormone auxin (DR5, GH3 and R2D2), cell identities, like protonema-specific proteins (RM09 and RM55) or mature rhizoids (RSL1,2), and developmental switches such as 2D-to-3D transition markers. In **Table 1**, references to all these reporters are indicated.

Visualised	Fusion/Target	Purpose	Reference
Nucleus	NLS4-GFP-GUS	Nuclear localisation	[21]
Endomembrane system		Endoplasmic reticulum	[11]
	α-1,2-mannosidase	Golgi apparatus imaging	[88]
	Targeting signal type 1 (SKL)	Peroxisome imaging	[88]
Mitochondria	Cytochrome c oxidase	Mitochondria imaging	[88]
Cytoskeleton	LifeAct	Actin cytoskeleton	[89]
	Tubulin α	Microtubule cytoskeleton	[90]
	MAP65	Antiparallel Microtubule-microtubule contacts	[91]
	Kinesins		[90]
Plasma membrane	SNAP-TM-mCherry	Membrane tracking	[21]
Auxin	pDR5v2:GFP-GUS	Aux. induced fluor.	[92]
	GH3:GFP-GUS	Aux. induced fluor.	
	R2D2	Ratiometric induction	
Protonema	pRM09:NLS4-GFP-GUS	Protonema identity reporting	[29]
	pRM55:NLS4-GFP-GUS	Protonema identity reporting	

Table 1.
Compilation of key molecular reporter lines published in literature to study cell and developmental processes in P. patens.

3.1.3 Microfluidics

Despite the advantageous physiological features of *P. patens*, observing cellular and subcellular processes with high resolution and for long periods of time is challenging. Traditionally, monitoring the intrinsic changes involved in regeneration, tip growth, bud formation, gametophore development and phyllid development, such as cytoskeleton organisation, protein distribution, organelle location, etc. has been done in glass-bottom petri dishes for as long as culture media could sustain, or in coverslip-sandwich sample preparations for up to few hours, due to lack of gas exchange [16, 37, 93–95]. However, the advent of microfluidics for bioimaging offers a new tool to overcome some limitations.

Microfluidic devices are transparent and flexible structures commonly produced using the biocompatible and air-permeable polydimethylsiloxane (PDMS) polymer. In biology, they have been used for study and imaging of cell and tissue development *in vivo*, including 3D development. For instance, it has been beneficial for high-throughput Arabidopsis root research [96]. Remarkably, the growth fashion of the pollen tube and the embryo development in Arabidopsis or the protonemal growth and early gametophore development of *P. patens* are ideal candidates for high-throughput and high-resolution imaging in microfluidic devices with light- and fluorescence-based microscopies [93, 97].

Until now, *P. patens*-tailored microfluidic devices have proven to be a reliable system for the monitoring of previously mentioned processes, as they offer tracking for up to weeks thanks to the air-permeability and possibility to refresh the media by circulating it from a reservoir [16]. Furthermore, it is then possible to introduce chemical agents or co-culture other organisms to image their cytological and gene expression effects on the plant over long periods of time [93]. The close tracking allows for quantitative cell measurements such as biomechanic parameters, growth rate and size of different tissues, frequency and geometry of divisions, developmental time and pace studies, etc. Microfluidic devices can capture subtle phenotypes of mutant lines for full analysis and high-quality phenotype reporting [16, 93].

3.2 Manipulation

3.2.1 Forward genetics

Some groups carried out forward genetic screening by X-ray or chemical mutagens that generated mutants with hormone resistance or abnormal tropic responses [85, 98]. However, due to the lack of genomic information, the disrupted genes that caused the phenotypes were never identified.

Recently, the completion of genome sequencing and the establishment of its genetic mapping tools removed the obstacles in the forward genetic screening of *P. patens*. To establish genetic mapping, two genetically divergent ecotypes of *P. patens*, Gransden and Villersexel were used [99].

With this genetic mapping resource, in the past few years, researchers started to perform forward genetic screening by treating protoplast with UV light. In such screenings, mutants with phenotypic defects were successfully obtained and the causal lesions were identified by outcrossing and whole genome sequencing. Notably, essential genes that are crucial for growth may not be identified due to the lethality of their knock-outs; therefore, conditional screening was performed to overcome this problem. After the UV light treatment, plants were cultured under different temperatures and in such conditions, plants showed growth defect only in high temperature were selected as a temperature-sensitive mutant [100].

Another screening aimed to discover genes that are essential for the 2D-to-3D transition is also limited by developmental defects, given that mutants in this process cannot produce gametophores necessary for sexual crossing. To overcome this problem, instead of crossing, researchers generated somatic hybrids between Villersexel mutants and Gransden wildtype, which produced diploid sporophytes [34]. Spores released from this hybrid sporophyte exhibited consistent phenotypic segregation ratio with meiosis. Mutant plants generated from these diploid spores were sequenced and genomically mapped to achieve the identification of new crucial genes for moss 2D-to-3D transition (e.g. NO GAMETOPHORES 1 and 2, or NOG1, NOG2).

In addition to UV light, tobacco Tnt1 retrotransposon was used to produce insertional mutations in genic and GC-rich regions [101]. Both PEG- or Agrobacterium-mediated transformations were applied and successfully produced mutants.

3.2.2 Gene identification

P. patens was the first moss fully sequenced. Organelle genomes were sequenced in 2003 (plastids) and 2007 (mitochondria) and nuclear genome in 2008, with the latest fully annotated revision made and genetic mapping obtained in 2018 [47]. This information and the molecular tools available allow targeted mutagenesis to dissect functions of genes of interest. Additionally, full genome structure and SNP variation between four main ecotypes (Gransden, Reute, Villersexel and Kaskaskia) was reported in 2017, completing the toolbox for reverse genetics and bioinformatics research.

3.2.3 Neutral locus integration

The integration of DNA constructs (including promoter, gene of interest and selection cassettes) necessary to produce transformants with stable expression and

Locus	Vector	Purpose	Reference
PIG1 locus	pGX8 pGG626	XVE inducible overexpression XVE inducible RNAi expression	[102, 103]
Pp108 locus	pUGGi	Constitutive RNAi expression	[104]
Pp108 locus	pTH-Ubi-Gate	Constitutive expression by the maize ubiquitin promoter	[105]
Redundant copy of the ARPC2 gene	pTK-Ubi-Gate		
Redundant copy of the ARPC3 gene	pTZ-Ubi-Gate		
PTA1 locus	pT10G	Overexpression by EF1α promoter	[106]
BS213 locus	pMJ1		[107]

Table 2.
A compilation of vectors designed to target proven neutral loci in P. patens.

non-disrupting phenotypes requires targeting of neutral loci that do not intrinsically produce a phenotype when disrupted, often due to gene redundancy. In **Table 2**, there are several standard neutral loci indicated which reportedly showed no visible phenotypes or morphological defects when it is replaced by an entire gene expression cassette.

Currently there are several vector sets released to specifically target neutral loci, that contain their flanking regions homologous to parts of the locus at start and end of the vector. Cloning the gene of interest in between readily allows replacement of the targeted locus with the entire cassette via homologous recombination (see section *Homologous recombination*).

In *P. patens*, the gene loci have three commonly seen annotations in literature. The first and standardised since 2017 (with the third chromosome annotation version) is PpGcX_uuyyyVn.m, where *G* is the genome release version (version 3), *c* stands for chromosome, *X* stands for chromosome number (from 1 to 27), and *uuyyy* is an arbitrary flexible number that indicates the exact locus; *V* stands for version, *n* for annotation version and *m* for locus version. Previous nomenclatures and equivalences can be found elsewhere [108]. In **Table 2**, loci are named as the original publication for traceability.

3.2.4 Homologous recombination

P. patens possesses an extremely high capacity of homologous recombination, which allows researchers to alter moss genomic DNA in any desired endogenous locus [14]. A common workflow is gene deletion by replacement with an antibiotic cassette. Also, protein localization studies with endogenous expression level is easily achieved by fusion of the fluorescent gene reporter sequence right after the target gene. Some vector sets for knock-out and knock-in to edit moss genome have been established and can be requested from several research groups (see **Table 2**) [11, 109]. Due to the ancestral genome duplication events in moss evolution, there is high functional redundancy of several gene families that decrease the risk of unwanted ortholog disruption.

3.2.5 Targeted double strand break and directed repair (CRISPR/Cas9)

The game-changing CRISPR/Cas9 method has proven an efficient and effective tool in *P. patens* to achieve large deletions, localised knock-in and point mutations [110, 111]. Transient transformation, flexibility of selection strategy and easy cloning workflow has rendered CRISPR/Cas9 transformation an established tool for

P. patens research. Two groups developed whole CRISPR/Cas9 platforms independently with high editing efficiencies.

In Nogué's lab, a co-delivery method was developed where each element of the system (Cas9, sgRNA and selection cassettes) was present in a separate plasmid. In this method, Cas9 expression is driven by an actin promoter and ready to use as is. The selection strategy can be chosen freely due to the lack of integration, minding the presence of resistance in the background lines. This method is also suitable for multiple mutations in different genes at once, given that more than one sgRNA plasmid can be simultaneously delivered in one transformation with still sufficiently high efficiencies of transformation [110].

In Bezanilla's lab, a whole set of gateway destination vectors for CRISPR/Cas9 system was developed. The strategy was to design a vector set to finally put all the three essential components (Cas9, sgRNA and selection cassettes) in a single expression plasmid. In both protocols, the sgRNA can be designed and optimised using the online design tool CRISPOR V1 against *P. patens* genome Phytozome V11 [112].

To increase the accuracy of mutations, the CRISPR/Cas9 system is applied with a homology-directed repair (HDR), which allows for seamless knock-in or point mutation in desired sites. The template DNA can be a donor plasmid that harbours homologous fragments or oligodeoxynucleotides (ODNs) [111, 113]. By co-transforming the plasmid or ODNs together with CRISPR/Cas9 and sgRNA vectors, both methods show high accuracy to generate a desired point mutation or scarless insertion with a fluorescence tag at any suitable location of the gene.

3.2.6 RNA interference

Given that moss possesses a relatively big gene family, arguably due to its double genome duplication, the employment of gene deletion strategies might be inefficient to investigate gene functions due to the high redundancy rate (e.g. there are four ROP genes with highly homologous or identical sequences) [38]. For this, RNA interference (RNAi) strategies offer an alternative to overcome this problem, and the procedure has been well-established.

To generate an RNAi construct for a gene of interest, a DNA sequence of 300 to 1000 bp is subcloned in a destination vector. After standard PEG-mediated transformation, the silencing effect can be detected after 24 h and last up to 3 weeks [104]. To avoid lethal effects when constitutively expressing interfering RNA, an oestradiol-inducible RNAi system is available [102]. Coupling RNAi silencing activation with fluorescent reporters facilitates screenings of loss of function phenotypes [104].

3.3 Transformation

Standard transformation protocols have been applicable to *P. patens* for a long time. In **Table 3**, three methods are shown, with key protocol references for their experimental application. The most essential step after transformation is phenotypic characterisation, that is often performed at the colony level (as it is derived from the microscopic phenotypes). Some phenotypes that must be compared with the reference wild type ecotype include colony size, shape, colour, texture, gametophore count and ratio of gametophore number to colony surface. In the microscopic level, protonemal parameters such as chloronema and caulonema cell length, thickness, growth rate and transition and ratio of one to the other are valuable indicators of several hormone and developmental processes. Naturally, the phenotyping should include characteristics associated to the process of study.

Strategy	Highlights	Reference
PEG/Mannitol	One to two round selection, 10% of transformants, 3–4 weeks for stable transformants	[114–117]
Agrobacterium tumefaciens	Four-round selection, 100% positive transformants, 12–16 weeks	[118]
Particle bombardment	Easy to conduct; less used. Transient and stable DNA integration.	[119]

Table 3.
Summary table of the classical and current transformation techniques and reference protocols for application.

4. Beyond *P. patens*

Due to their accessibility, tractability and close yet independent phylogenetic position, the interest in Bryophytes has increased dramatically in the last decade [1]. Beyond *P. patens*, mosses have garnered special interest for their physiology and development, involvement in carbon sequestration, abiotic stresses management and biotic interactions. Eight species have had their nuclear genome sequenced and drafted in the last few years, and at least thirteen others are currently being sequenced [120–127]. Furthermore, the mitochondrial and/or plastid genomes of more than forty other moss species (not cited) has been published in the last six years, which may precede their nuclear genome study as with *P. patens*. This level of knowledge is an essential tool to dissect the molecular basis of processes under study, and the recent and future increase in the availability of this information is going to dramatically accelerate research in mosses, among other bryophytes [128]. In this section, a collection of mosses at the frontier of moss cell and molecular research are highlighted for their ecological relevance, distinct physiology and genetic composition, among others. We believe these will be the next generation of mosses for research that will provide new insights in plant research beyond *P. patens* in the coming years.

4.1 *Ceratodon purpureus* (Hedw.) Brid.

The fire moss *C. purpureus* (Dicranales, Bryopsida) is a cosmopolitan species that thrives in diverse ecosystems, including hostile post-wildfire or heavy metal-contaminated areas, and those with high radiation and freezing temperatures [129, 130]. The life cycle of this moss involves male and female haploid individuals due to the presence of sexual chromosomes. Consequently, it has become a reference for dioecious reproduction and sexual dimorphism, with some developmental differences in sexual and non-sexual features [131, 132]. In 2021, male and female nuclear annotated genomes were published, making *Ceratodon* the third sequenced moss genus [127]. Furthermore, gene targeting in this species has been proven effective, providing all the basic tools for cell and molecular biology research [133]. Importantly, the similarity of growth fashion between *C. purpureus* and *P. patens* will provide a new reference to study the discussed developmental processes in higher depth.

4.2 Hypnales W.R. Buck & Vitt

The Hypnales (Bryopsida) are the biggest and most diverse order of mosses with varied morphology, and mostly exhibit pleurocarpous (i.e. non-erect) growth fashion. It includes *Fontinalis antipyretica* Hedw., *Pleurozium schreberi* (Brid.) Mitt. and *Calohypnum plumiforme* (Wilson) Kučera & Ignatov, the genome sequences of which have been published in the last two years [123, 125, 134]. *P. schreberi* is attractive due to its documented symbiotic relationships with N_2-fixing cyanobacteria and *C. plumiforme* for bryophyte-exclusive biosynthetic gene clusters research [123, 134]. As pleurocarps, all of them exhibit a non-erect plant architecture that suggests an adapted regulation of stem development.

Remarkably, the common aquatic moss *F. antipyretica* is a globally distributed species and serves as a reference organism for the study of land-to-water habitat reversal and its genetic basis. From the developmental processes' perspective, this moss has a distinct interest due to its tristichous phyllotactic pattern (120° rotation from organ to organ) that can serve as a reference in the investigation of genetic regulation of asymmetric cell divisions in the shoot apical cell at the gametophore apex (see **Figure 1**) [24].

4.3 *Sphagnum* L.

The genus *Sphagnum* (Sphagnales, Sphagnopsida) plays an important ecological role in the climate change situation, as its species are important carbon fixators. For this reason, The Sphagnome Project was created in 2018 in the aim to sequence fifteen species across the genus [124]. At this moment, the genomes of *Sphagnum fallax* and *Sphagnum magellanicum* have been published [124]. From the developmental point of view, *Sphagnum* spp. are attractive due to their branching gametophores and subsequent implications in lateral shoot meristems and phyllotaxis, which is different from *P. patens* and *C. purpureus*. Furthermore, *Sphagnum spp.* do not show rhizoids and some species are mostly or fully aquatic, serving as models for land-to-water reversal. Remarkably, *Sphagnum* spp. do not develop filamentous protonemata as most mosses, but thalloid protonemata (i.e. disk-like, bidimensional), as that of liverworts [135].

4.4 Polytrichopsida Doweld

The moss class Polytrichopsida is the second biggest (~200 species) after Bryopsida (~11500 species), and its species have unique morphological characteristics that make them uniquely interesting for developmental biology [5]. Despite mosses being regarded as avascular plants, some exhibit hydroids and leptoids, a functionally analogous tissue to tracheids and sieve elements of vascular plants that slightly differs morphologically and developmentally. Polytrichopsida has several genera with such structures, in some cases underdeveloped and, in others, completely functional, like in *Polytrichum* and *Dawsonia*, with up to 65-cm tall gametophores [5, 136]. This distinct characteristic suggests that xylem-like structures evolved independently and thus the genetic and molecular machinery necessary to its development may have similar origins to that of fern, gymnosperm, and angiosperm vasculature. Another attractive feature of several genera of Polytrichaceae is the perpendicular lamellae on the unistratose phyllids, that represents an increase in leaf complexity and has proven to be an alternative evolutionary path for increased photosynthetic capacity.

Despite its potential to provide valuable insight, genetic tools have barely been developed for this taxon, but full mitochondrial and plastid genomes have recently been published for *Polytrichum commune*, a cosmopolitan species ~10 cm long that has a complete stem vasculature [137, 138].

4.5 Other mosses

The desert moss *Syntrichia caninervis* Mitt. (Pottiales, Bryopsida) is the first outstanding example of dessication-tolerant moss to have its genome sequenced [126].

This genome will provide tools to dissect the development of the unique sub-micron structures of its phyllids that stimulate water capture and what genes are involved in the asymmetric growth and divisions necessary for this structure [139].

The heavy metal-tolerant moss *Scopelophila cataratae* (Mitt.) Broth. (Pottiales, Bryopsida), capable of thriving in copper-rich environments, has had its genome drafted (unpublished, 2016) and CRISPR/Cas9 mutagenesis demonstrated [121].

Funaria hygrometrica Hedw. (Funariales, Bryopsida) is evolutionary close to *P. patens*, and they have virtually identical morphology at the gametophyte generation, but remarkably different sporophyte generation. *F. hygrometrica* has a longer seta, different mechanisms and regulation of spore release [140]. However, the level of difference in their transcriptome is unexpectedly high and transcripts seem to be shifted in expression time but not in sequence. The recently published genome may allow investigate how time-shifted expression of regulators impacts morphology [120].

5. Conclusions

We have shown how mosses are an increasingly relevant model group to plant developmental biology due to their distinct accessibility at physiological and molecular level. Their evolutionary distance with agronomically relevant plants does not diminish their potential to help to understand fundamental questions of development that remain unsolved, given that most essential regulatory networks are conserved. This has been shown in the hormonal regulation of branching and shoot and root development, regeneration, the establishment of shoot apical cells and the genetic make-up in 2D-to-3D transition. The utility of mosses has convinced the scientific community to the point of promoting the sequencing of eight new species to explore other physiological processes in the last few years. We have also shown how *Physcomitrium patens* is a workhorse in cell and molecular biology of plants, and provided evidence that it is likely to become a standard tool of plant developmental biology together with a number of other mosses.

Acknowledgements

The authors would like to thank Dr. Jeroen de Keijzer and Dr. Tijs Ketelaar for their thoughtful and detailed review of the manuscript. Also, the funding agencies Technology, Knowledge and Innovation, division Horticulture and Propagating Material (TKI T&U) and the Dutch Research Council (NWO) (reference number: TKILWV20.390) for funding JFC and the ERC grant to Prof. J. Friml (reference number: PR1023ERC02) for funding HT. The authors would like to sincerely apologise for the literature not cited that may be relevant for this chapter and is not present due to space constraints.

Author details

Jordi Floriach-Clark[1], Han Tang[2] and Viola Willemsen[1*]

1 Wageningen University, Wageningen, The Netherlands

2 Institute of Science and Technology Austria, Klosterneuburg, Austria

*Address all correspondence to: viola.willemsen@wur.nl

References

[1] Cheng S, Xian W, Fu Y, Marin B, Keller J, Wu T, et al. Genomes of Subaerial Zygnematophyceae Provide Insights into Land Plant Evolution. Cell. 2019;179(5):1057-1067.e14.

[2] McDaniel SF. Bryophytes are not early diverging land plants. New Phytol. 2021;230(4):1300-4.

[3] Green TGA, Clayton-Greene KA. Studies on Dawsonia superba Grev. II. Growth rate. J Bryol. 1981;11(4):723-31.

[4] Medina NG, Draper I, Lara F. Biogeography of mosses and allies: does size matter? In: Fontaneto D, editor. Biogeography of Microscopic Organisms: Is Everything Small Everywhere? [Internet]. Cambridge: Cambridge University Press; 2011. p. 209-33. (Systematics Association Special Volume Series). Available from: https://www.cambridge.org/core/books/biogeography-of-microscopic-organisms/biogeography-of-mosses-and-allies-does-size-matter/11003DB9B3BC0FE5CF5F603BFB4AF4A1

[5] Bell N, Kariyawasam I, Flores J, Hyvönen J. The diversity of the Polytrichopsida—a review. Bryophyt Divers Evol [Internet]. 2021 Jun 30 [cited 2021 Sep 7];043(1):98-111. Available from: https://www.biotaxa.org/dbe/article/view/bde.43.1.8

[6] Ekwealor JTB, Fisher KM. Life under quartz: Hypolithic mosses in the Mojave Desert. PLoS One [Internet]. 2020 [cited 2021 Jul 28];15(7):e0235928. Available from: https://journals.plos.org/plosone/article?id=10.1371/journal.pone.0235928

[7] Górski P, Gądek B, Gąbka M. Snow as a parameter of bryophyte niche partitioning in snow-beds of the Tatra Mountains (Western Carpathians). Ecol Indic. 2020 Jun 1;113:106258.

[8] Nakosteen PC, Hughes KW. Sexual Life Cycle of Three Species of Funariaceae in Culture. Bryologist [Internet]. 1978 Aug 31;81(2):307-14. Available from: https://www.jstor.org/stable/3242191

[9] Reski R. Quantitative moss cell biology. Curr Opin Plant Biol. 2018 Dec 1;46:39-47.

[10] Xu B, Ohtani M, Yamaguchi M, Toyooka K, Wakazaki M, Sato M, et al. Contribution of NAC transcription factors to plant adaptation to land. Science (80-). 2014;343(6178):1505-8.

[11] Rensing SA, Goffinet B, Meyberg R, Wu S-ZZ, Bezanilla M. The moss physcomitrium (Physcomitrella) patens: A model organism for non-seed plants. Plant Cell [Internet]. 2020 May 1 [cited 2021 Jun 16];32(5):1361-76. Available from: www.plantcell.org/cgi/doi/10.1105/tpc.19.00828

[12] de Keijzer J, Rios AF, Willemsen V. Physcomitrium patens: A single model to study oriented cell divisions in 1d to 3d patterning. Int J Mol Sci [Internet]. 2021 Mar 1 [cited 2021 Jun 16];22(5): 1-16. Available from: https://doi.org/10.3390/ijms22052626

[13] Perroud P-F, Meyberg R, Demko V, Quatrano RS, Olsen O-A, Rensing SA. DEK1 displays a strong subcellular polarity during *Physcomitrella patens* 3D growth. New Phytol [Internet]. 2020 May 1 [cited 2021 Aug 4];226(4):1029-41. Available from: https://nph-onlinelibrary-wiley-com.ezproxy.library.wur.nl/doi/full/10.1111/nph.16417

[14] Prigge MJ, Bezanilla M. Evolutionary crossroads in developmental biology: *Physcomitrella patens*. Development. 2010 Nov 1;137(21):3535-43.

[15] Hoffmann B, Proust H, Belcram K, Labrune C, Boyer F-D, Rameau C, et al. Strigolactones Inhibit Caulonema Elongation and Cell Division in the Moss *Physcomitrella patens*. PLoS One [Internet]. 2014 Jun 9 [cited 2021 Sep 2];9(6):e99206. Available from: https://journals.plos.org/plosone/article?id=10.1371/journal.pone.0099206

[16] Bascom CS, Wu S-Z, Nelson K, Oakey J, Bezanilla M. Long-Term Growth of Moss in Microfluidic Devices Enables Subcellular Studies in Development. Plant Physiol [Internet]. 2016 Sep 1 [cited 2021 Jun 17];172(1):28-37. Available from: https://academic.oup.com/plphys/article/172/1/28-37/6115611

[17] Cove DJ, Knight CD, Lamparter T. Mosses as model systems. Trends Plant Sci [Internet]. 1997 Mar 1 [cited 2021 Sep 2];2(3):99-105. Available from: http://www.cell.com/article/S136013859610056X/fulltext

[18] Jaeger R, Moody LA. A fundamental developmental transition in Physcomitrium patens is regulated by evolutionarily conserved mechanisms [Internet]. Vol. 23, Evolution and Development. Blackwell Publishing Inc.; 2021 [cited 2021 Jun 16]. p. 123-36. Available from: https://onlinelibrary.wiley.com/doi/full/10.1111/ede.12376

[19] Thelander M, Olsson T, Ronne H. Effect of the energy supply on filamentous growth and development in *Physcomitrella patens*. J Exp Bot [Internet]. 2005 Feb 1 [cited 2021 Sep 2];56(412):653-62. Available from: https://academic.oup.com/jxb/article/56/412/653/580262

[20] Moody LA. The 2D to 3D growth transition in the moss *Physcomitrella patens*. Curr Opin Plant Biol [Internet]. 2019 Feb 1 [cited 2021 Aug 5];47:88-95. Available from: https://doi.org/10.1016/j.pbi.2018.10.001

[21] Tang H, Duijts K, Bezanilla M, Scheres B, Vermeer JEM, Willemsen V. Geometric cues forecast the switch from two- to three-dimensional growth in *Physcomitrella patens*. New Phytol. 2020;225(5):1945-55.

[22] Sakakibara K, Nishiyama T, Sumikawa N, Kofuji R, Murata T, Hasebe M. Involvement of auxin and a homeodomain-leucine zipper I gene in rhizoid development of the moss *Physcomitrella patens*. Development. 2003 Oct 15;130(20):4835-46.

[23] Jang G, Yi K, Pires ND, Menand B, Dolan L. RSL genes are sufficient for rhizoid system development in early diverging land plants. Development [Internet]. 2011 Jun 1 [cited 2021 Aug 31];138(11):2273-81. Available from: http://mrbayes.csit.fsu.edu/

[24] Véron E, Vernoux T, Coudert Y. Phyllotaxis from a Single Apical Cell. Trends Plant Sci [Internet]. 2021 Feb 1 [cited 2021 Jun 16];26(2):124-31. Available from: https://doi.org/10.1016/j.tplants.2020.09.014

[25] Hohe A, Rensing SA, Mildner M, Lang D, Reski R. Day Length and Temperature Strongly Influence Sexual Reproduction and Expression of a Novel MADS-Box Gene in the Moss *Physcomitrella patens*. Plant Biol [Internet]. 2002 Sep 1 [cited 2021 Aug 31];4(5):595-602. Available from: https://onlinelibrary.wiley.com/doi/full/10.1055/s-2002-35440

[26] Hiss M, Meyberg R, Westermann J, Haas FB, Schneider L, Schallenberg-Rüdinger M, et al. Sexual reproduction, sporophyte development and molecular variation in the model moss *Physcomitrella patens*: introducing the ecotype Reute. Plant J [Internet]. 2017 May 1 [cited 2021 Jul 27];90(3):606-20. Available from: https://onlinelibrary.wiley.com/doi/full/10.1111/tpj.13501

[27] Meyberg R, Perroud P-F, Haas FB, Schneider L, Heimerl T, Renzaglia KS, et al. Characterisation of evolutionarily conserved key players affecting eukaryotic flagellar motility and fertility using a moss model. New Phytol [Internet]. 2020 Jul 1 [cited 2021 Jul 28];227(2):440-54. Available from: https://nph.onlinelibrary.wiley.com/doi/full/10.1111/nph.16486

[28] Cervantes-Pérez D, Ortega-García A, Medina-Andrés R, Batista-García RA, Lira-Ruan V. Exogenous Nitric Oxide Delays Plant Regeneration from Protoplast and Protonema Development in *Physcomitrella patens*. Plants 2020, Vol 9, Page 1380 [Internet]. 2020 Oct 16 [cited 2021 Jul 28];9(10):1380. Available from: https://www.mdpi.com/2223-7747/9/10/1380/htm

[29] Ishikawa M, Murata T, Sato Y, Nishiyama T, Hiwatashi Y, Imai A, et al. Physcomitrella Cyclin-Dependent Kinase A Links Cell Cycle Reactivation to Other Cellular Changes during Reprogramming of Leaf Cells. Plant Cell [Internet]. 2011 Aug 1 [cited 2021 Jul 28];23(8):2924-38. Available from: https://academic.oup.com/plcell/article/23/8/2924/6097203

[30] KNIGHT CD, COVE DJ. The polarity of gravitropism in the moss *Physcomitrella patens* is reversed during mitosis and after growth on a clinostat. Plant Cell Environ [Internet]. 1991 Dec 1 [cited 2021 Aug 31];14(9):995-1001. Available from: https://onlinelibrary.wiley.com/doi/full/10.1111/j.1365-3040.1991.tb00970.x

[31] Jenkins GI, Cove DJ. Phototropism and polarotropism of primary chloronemata of the moss *Physcomitrella patens*: responses of mutant strains. Planta 1983 1595 [Internet]. 1983 Nov [cited 2021 Aug 31];159(5):432-8. Available from: https://link.springer.com/article/10.1007/BF00392079

[32] Bao L, Yamamoto KT, Fujita T. Phototropism in gametophytic shoots of the moss *Physcomitrella patens*. Plant Signal Behav [Internet]. 2015 Apr 7 [cited 2021 Aug 31];10(3). Available from: https://www.tandfonline.com/doi/abs/10.1080/15592324.2015.1010900

[33] Harrison CJ, Roeder AHK, Meyerowitz EM, Langdale JA. Local Cues and Asymmetric Cell Divisions Underpin Body Plan Transitions in the Moss *Physcomitrella patens*. Curr Biol. 2009 Mar 24;19(6):461-71.

[34] Moody LA, Kelly S, Rabbinowitsch E, Langdale JA. Genetic Regulation of the 2D to 3D Growth Transition in the Moss *Physcomitrella patens*. Curr Biol. 2018 Feb 5;28(3):473-478.e5.

[35] Perroud P-F, Demko V, Johansen W, Wilson RC, Olsen O-A, Quatrano RS. Defective Kernel 1 (DEK1) is required for three-dimensional growth in *Physcomitrella patens*. New Phytol [Internet]. 2014 Aug 1 [cited 2021 Jul 28];203(3):794-804. Available from: https://nph-onlinelibrary-wiley-com.ezproxy.library.wur.nl/doi/full/10.1111/nph.12844

[36] Moody LA, Kelly S, Clayton R, Weeks Z, Emms DM, Langdale JA. NO GAMETOPHORES 2 Is a Novel Regulator of the 2D to 3D Growth Transition in the Moss *Physcomitrella patens*. Curr Biol. 2021 Feb 8;31(3):555-563.e4.

[37] Yi P, Goshima G. Rho of Plants GTPases and Cytoskeletal Elements Control Nuclear Positioning and Asymmetric Cell Division during *Physcomitrella patens* Branching. Curr Biol [Internet]. 2020;30(14):2860-2868.e3. Available from: https://doi.org/10.1016/j.cub.2020.05.022

[38] Cheng X, Mwaura BW, Chang Stauffer SR, Bezanilla M. A Fully Functional ROP Fluorescent Fusion

Protein Reveals Roles for This GTPase in Subcellular and Tissue-Level Patterning. Plant Cell [Internet]. 2020 Nov 2 [cited 2021 Aug 11];32(11):3436-51. Available from: https://academic.oup.com/plcell/article/32/11/3436/6099412

[39] Kimata Y, Higaki T, Kawashima T, Kurihara D, Sato Y, Yamada T, et al. Cytoskeleton dynamics control the first asymmetric cell division in Arabidopsis zygote. Proc Natl Acad Sci [Internet]. 2016 Dec 6 [cited 2021 Sep 1];113(49):14157-62. Available from: https://www.pnas.org/content/113/49/14157

[40] Sussex IM, Kerk NM. The evolution of plant architecture. Curr Opin Plant Biol. 2001 Feb 1;4(1):33-7.

[41] Shi B, Vernoux T. Patterning at the shoot apical meristem and phyllotaxis. Curr Top Dev Biol. 2019 Jan 1;131:81-107.

[42] Barton MK. Twenty years on: The inner workings of the shoot apical meristem, a developmental dynamo. Dev Biol. 2010 May 1;341(1):95-113.

[43] Harrison CJ. Development and genetics in the evolution of land plant body plans. Philos Trans R Soc B Biol Sci [Internet]. 2017 Feb 5 [cited 2021 Aug 23];372(1713). Available from: https://royalsocietypublishing.org/doi/abs/10.1098/rstb.2015.0490

[44] Hata Y, Kyozuka J. Fundamental mechanisms of the stem cell regulation in land plants: lesson from shoot apical cells in bryophytes. Plant Mol Biol 2021 [Internet]. 2021 Feb 20 [cited 2021 Aug 23];1:1-13. Available from: https://link.springer.com/article/10.1007/s11103-021-01126-y

[45] Haig D. Homologous Versus Antithetic Alternation of Generations and the Origin of Sporophytes. Bot Rev 2008 743 [Internet]. 2008 Jul 26 [cited 2021 Aug 23];74(3):395-418. Available from: https://link-springer-com.ezproxy.library.wur.nl/article/10.1007/s12229-008-9012-x

[46] Bennici A. Origin and early evolution of land plants. http://www-tandfonline-com.ezproxy.library.wur.nl/action/authorSubmission?journalCode=kcib20&page=instructions [Internet]. 2008 Oct [cited 2021 Sep 12];1(2):212-8. Available from: https://www-tandfonline-com.ezproxy.library.wur.nl/doi/abs/10.4161/cib.1.2.6987

[47] Rensing SA, Lang D, Zimmer AD, Terry A, Salamov A, Shapiro H, et al. The Physcomitrella Genome Reveals Evolutionary Insights into the Conquest of Land by Plants. Science (80-) [Internet]. 2008 Jan 4 [cited 2021 Aug 23];319(5859):64-9. Available from: https://science-sciencemag-org.ezproxy.library.wur.nl/content/319/5859/64

[48] Frank MH, Scanlon MJ. Cell-specific transcriptomic analyses of three-dimensional shoot development in the moss *Physcomitrella patens*. Plant J [Internet]. 2015 Aug 1 [cited 2021 Aug 23];83(4):743-51. Available from: https://onlinelibrary.wiley.com/doi/full/10.1111/tpj.12928

[49] Hofmeister W. Allgemeine Morphologie der Gewächse. Leipzig; 1868. 259 p.

[50] Givnish TJ. Ecological constraints on the evolution of plasticity in plants. Evol Ecol 2002 163 [Internet]. 2002 [cited 2021 Sep 15];16(3):213-42. Available from: https://link.springer.com/article/10.1023/A:1019676410041

[51] Bravais L, Bravais A. Essai sur la disposition des feuilles curvisériées. Annales des sciences naturelles (Botanique); 1837. 69 p.

[52] Gola EM, Banasiak A. Diversity of phyllotaxis in land plants in reference to the shoot apical meristem structure. Acta Soc Bot Pol [Internet]. 2016 Dec 31 [cited 2021 Aug 24];85(4). Available

from: https://pbsociety.org.pl/journals/index.php/asbp/article/view/6873

[53] Jean R V. Phyllotaxis: A Systemic Study in Plant Morphogenesis [Internet]. Cambridge: Cambridge University Press; 1994. 401 p. Available from: https://www.cambridge.org/core/books/phyllotaxis/272D9010BE175D26B61D5A2ED8D87A3C

[54] Moody LA. Three-dimensional growth: a developmental innovation that facilitated plant terrestrialization. J Plant Res 2020 1333 [Internet]. 2020 Feb 24 [cited 2021 Aug 4];133(3):283-90. Available from: https://link-springer-com.ezproxy.library.wur.nl/article/10.1007/s10265-020-01173-4

[55] Kamamoto N, Tano T, Fujimoto K, Shimamura M. Rotation angle of stem cell division plane controls spiral phyllotaxis in mosses. J Plant Res [Internet]. 2021 May 1 [cited 2021 Jun 16];134(3):457-73. Available from: https://doi.org/10.1007/s10265-021-01298-0

[56] Zagórska-Marek B, Sokołowska K, Turzańska M. Chiral events in developing gametophores of *Physcomitrella patens* and other moss species are driven by an unknown, universal direction-sensing mechanism. Am J Bot [Internet]. 2018 Dec 1 [cited 2021 Aug 24];105(12):1986-94. Available from: https://bsapubs.onlinelibrary.wiley.com/doi/full/10.1002/ajb2.1200

[57] Xu L. De novo root regeneration from leaf explants: wounding, auxin, and cell fate transition. Curr Opin Plant Biol. 2018 Feb 1;41:39-45.

[58] Mathew MM, Prasad K. Model systems for regeneration: Arabidopsis. Development [Internet]. 2021 Mar 15 [cited 2021 Sep 2];148(6). Available from: https://dev.biologists.org/collection/

[59] Sato Y, Sugimoto N, Hirai T, Imai A, Kubo M, Hiwatashi Y, et al. Cells reprogramming to stem cells inhibit the reprogramming of adjacent cells in the moss *Physcomitrella patens*. Sci Reports 2017 71 [Internet]. 2017 May 15 [cited 2021 Jul 28];7(1):1-12. Available from: https://www.nature.com/articles/s41598-017-01786-1

[60] Ikeuchi M, Ogawa Y, Iwase A, Sugimoto K. Plant regeneration: Cellular origins and molecular mechanisms. Dev. 2016 May 1;143(9):1442-51.

[61] Kofuji R, Hasebe M. Eight types of stem cells in the life cycle of the moss *Physcomitrella patens*. Curr Opin Plant Biol. 2014 Feb 1;17(1):13-21.

[62] Ikeuchi M, Favero DS, Sakamoto Y, Iwase A, Coleman D, Rymen B, et al. Molecular Mechanisms of Plant Regeneration. Annu Rev Plant Biol [Internet]. 2019 Apr 29 [cited 2021 Sep 2];70(1):377-406. Available from: https://www.annualreviews.org/doi/10.1146/annurev-arplant-050718-100434

[63] Kubo M, Nishiyama T, Tamada Y, Sano R, Ishikawa M, Murata T, et al. Single-cell transcriptome analysis of Physcomitrella leaf cells during reprogramming using microcapillary manipulation. Nucleic Acids Res [Internet]. 2019 May 21 [cited 2021 Aug 24];47(9):4539-53. Available from: https://academic.oup.com/nar/article/47/9/4539/5381068

[64] Nishiyama T, Miyawaki K, Ohshima M, Thompson K, Nagashima A, Hasebe M, et al. Digital Gene Expression Profiling by 5′-End Sequencing of cDNAs during Reprogramming in the Moss *Physcomitrella patens*. PLoS One [Internet]. 2012 May 4 [cited 2021 Aug 24];7(5):e36471. Available from: https://journals.plos.org/plosone/article?id=10.1371/journal.pone.0036471

[65] Zhou W, Lozano-Torres JL, Blilou I, Zhang X, Zhai Q, Smant G, et al. A Jasmonate Signaling Network Activates

Root Stem Cells and Promotes Regeneration. Cell. 2019 May 2;177(4):942-956.e14.

[66] Kareem A, Durgaprasad K, Sugimoto K, Du Y, Pulianmackal AJ, Trivedi ZB, et al. PLETHORA genes control regeneration by a two-step mechanism. Curr Biol [Internet]. 2015;25(8):1017-30. Available from: http://dx.doi.org/10.1016/j.cub.2015.02.022

[67] Subban P, Kutsher Y, Evenor D, Belausov E, Zemach H, Faigenboim A, et al. Shoot Regeneration Is Not a Single Cell Event. Plants 2021, Vol 10, Page 58 [Internet]. 2020 Dec 29 [cited 2021 Sep 2];10(1):58. Available from: https://www.mdpi.com/2223-7747/10/1/58/htm

[68] Sakakibara K, Reisewitz P, Aoyama T, Friedrich T, Ando S, Sato Y, et al. WOX13-like genes are required for reprogramming of leaf and protoplast cells into stem cells in the moss *Physcomitrella patens*. Development. 2014 Apr 15;141(8):1660-70.

[69] Li C, Sako Y, Imai A, Nishiyama T, Thompson K, Kubo M, et al. A Lin28 homologue reprograms differentiated cells to stem cells in the moss *Physcomitrella patens*. Nat Commun 2017 81 [Internet]. 2017 Jan 27 [cited 2021 Aug 24];8(1):1-13. Available from: https://www.nature.com/articles/ncomms14242

[70] Ishikawa M, Morishita M, Higuchi Y, Ichikawa S, Ishikawa T, Nishiyama T, et al. Physcomitrella STEMIN transcription factor induces stem cell formation with epigenetic reprogramming. Nat Plants 2019 57 [Internet]. 2019 Jul 8 [cited 2021 Aug 24];5(7):681-90. Available from: https://www.nature.com/articles/s41477-019-0464-2

[71] Storti M, Costa A, Golin S, Zottini M, Morosinotto T, Alboresi A. Systemic Calcium Wave Propagation in *Physcomitrella patens*. Plant Cell Physiol [Internet]. 2018 Jul 1 [cited 2021 Aug 24];59(7):1377-84. Available from: https://academic.oup.com/pcp/article/59/7/1377/5033790

[72] Kleist TJ, Cartwright HN, Perera AM, Christianson ML, Lemaux PG, Luan S. Genetically encoded calcium indicators for fluorescence imaging in the moss Physcomitrella: GCaMP3 provides a bright new look. Plant Biotechnol J. 2017 Oct 1;15(10):1235-7.

[73] Nicolas WJ, Grison MS, Bayer EM. Shaping intercellular channels of plasmodesmata: the structure-to-function missing link. J Exp Bot [Internet]. 2018 Jan 1 [cited 2021 Aug 24];69(1):91-103. Available from: https://academic.oup.com/jxb/article/69/1/91/4107278

[74] Kitagawa M, Fujita T. Quantitative imaging of directional transport through plasmodesmata in moss protonemata via single-cell photoconversion of Dendra2. J Plant Res 2013 1264 [Internet]. 2013 Feb 5 [cited 2021 Aug 24];126(4):577-85. Available from: https://link.springer.com/article/10.1007/s10265-013-0547-5

[75] Kitagawa M, Tomoi T, Fukushima T, Sakata Y, Sato M, Toyooka K, et al. Abscisic Acid Acts as a Regulator of Molecular Trafficking through Plasmodesmata in the Moss *Physcomitrella patens*. Plant Cell Physiol [Internet]. 2019 Apr 1 [cited 2021 Aug 24];60(4):738-51. Available from: https://academic.oup.com/pcp/article/60/4/738/5267838

[76] Reinhardt D, Mandel T, Kuhlemeier C. Auxin Regulates the Initiation and Radial Position of Plant Lateral Organs. Plant Cell. 2000 Apr;12(4):507.

[77] Vanneste S, Friml J. Auxin: A Trigger for Change in Plant

Development. Cell. 2009 Mar 20;136(6):1005-16.

[78] MJ P, M L, NW A, M E. Physcomitrella patens auxin-resistant mutants affect conserved elements of an auxin-signaling pathway. Curr Biol [Internet]. 2010 Nov 9 [cited 2021 Sep 2];20(21):1907-12. Available from: https://pubmed.ncbi.nlm.nih.gov/20951049/

[79] Paponov IA, Teale W, Lang D, Paponov M, Reski R, Rensing SA, et al. The evolution of nuclear auxin signalling. BMC Evol Biol 2009 91 [Internet]. 2009 Jun 3 [cited 2021 Sep 2];9(1):1-16. Available from: https://bmcecolevol.biomedcentral.com/articles/10.1186/1471-2148-9-126

[80] Lavy M, Prigge MJ, Tao S, Shain S, Kuo A, Kirchsteiger K, et al. Constitutive auxin response in Physcomitrella reveals complex interactions between Aux/IAA and ARF proteins. Elife. 2016 Jun 1;5(JUN2016).

[81] TA B, MM L, T A, NM B, M B, Y C, et al. Plasma membrane-targeted PIN proteins drive shoot development in a moss. Curr Biol [Internet]. 2014 Dec 1 [cited 2021 Sep 2];24(23):2776-85. Available from: https://pubmed.ncbi.nlm.nih.gov/25448003/

[82] Viaene T, Landberg K, Thelander M, Medvecka E, Pederson E, Feraru E, et al. Directional Auxin Transport Mechanisms in Early Diverging Land Plants. Curr Biol. 2014 Dec 1;24(23):2786-91.

[83] Coudert Y, Palubicki W, Ljung K, Novak O, Leyser O, Harrison CJ. Three ancient hormonal cues co-ordinate shoot branching in a moss. Elife. 2015;4.

[84] Zürcher E, Tavor-Deslex D, Lituiev D, Enkerli K, Tarr PT, Müller B. A Robust and Sensitive Synthetic Sensor to Monitor the Transcriptional Output of the Cytokinin Signaling Network in Planta. Plant Physiol [Internet]. 2013 Feb 28 [cited 2021 Sep 15];161(3):1066-75. Available from: https://academic.oup.com/plphys/article/161/3/1066/6110587

[85] Ashton NW, Grimsley NH, Cove DJ. Analysis of Gametophytic Development in the Moss, *Physcomitrella patens*, Using Auxin and Cytokinin Resistant Mutants. Planta. 1933;435(5):1-46.

[86] Hyoung S, Cho SH, Chung JH, So WM, Cui MH, Shin JS. Cytokinin oxidase PpCKX1 plays regulatory roles in development and enhances dehydration and salt tolerance in *Physcomitrella patens*. Plant Cell Reports 2019 393 [Internet]. 2019 Dec 20 [cited 2021 Sep 15];39(3):419-30. Available from: https://link.springer.com/article/10.1007/s00299-019-02500-3

[87] Proust H, Hoffmann B, Xie X, Yoneyama K, Schaefer DG, Yoneyama K, et al. Strigolactones regulate protonema branching and act as a quorum sensing-like signal in the moss *Physcomitrella patens*. Development [Internet]. 2011 Apr 15 [cited 2021 Sep 16];138(8):1531-9. Available from: http://rsb.info.nih.gov/ij/

[88] Furt F, Lemoi K, Tüzel E, Vidali L. Quantitative analysis of organelle distribution and dynamics in *Physcomitrella patens* protonemal cells. BMC Plant Biol 2012 121 [Internet]. 2012 May 17 [cited 2021 Aug 24];12(1):1-15. Available from: https://bmcplantbiol.biomedcentral.com/articles/10.1186/1471-2229-12-70

[89] Vidali L, Gisbergen PAC van, Guérin C, Franco P, Li M, Burkart GM, et al. Rapid formin-mediated actin-filament elongation is essential for polarized plant cell growth. Proc Natl Acad Sci [Internet]. 2009 Aug 11 [cited 2021 Aug 24];106(32):13341-6. Available from: https://www.pnas.org/content/106/32/13341

[90] Hiwatashi Y, Obara M, Sato Y, Fujita T, Murata T, Hasebe M. Kinesins Are Indispensable for Interdigitation of Phragmoplast Microtubules in the Moss *Physcomitrella patens*. Plant Cell [Internet]. 2008 Dec 31 [cited 2021 Sep 2];20(11):3094-106. Available from: https://academic.oup.com/plcell/article/20/11/3094/6092527

[91] Kosetsu K, de Keijzer J, Janson ME, Goshima G. MICROTUBULE-ASSOCIATED PROTEIN65 Is Essential for Maintenance of Phragmoplast Bipolarity and Formation of the Cell Plate in *Physcomitrella patens*. Plant Cell [Internet]. 2013 Dec 30 [cited 2021 Aug 24];25(11):4479-92. Available from: https://academic.oup.com/plcell/article/25/11/4479/6096775

[92] Thelander M, Landberg K, Sundberg E. Minimal auxin sensing levels in vegetative moss stem cells revealed by a ratiometric reporter. New Phytol. 2019;224(2):775-88.

[93] Kozgunova E, Goshima G. A versatile microfluidic device for highly inclined thin illumination microscopy in the moss *Physcomitrella patens*. Sci Rep [Internet]. 2019 Dec 1 [cited 2021 Jun 17];9(1):1-8. Available from: https://doi.org/10.1038/s41598-019-51624-9

[94] Leong SY, Edzuka T, Goshima G, Yamada M. Kinesin-13 and Kinesin-8 Function during Cell Growth and Division in the Moss *Physcomitrella patens*. Plant Cell [Internet]. 2020 Mar 2 [cited 2021 Aug 3];32(3):683-702. Available from: https://academic-oup-com.ezproxy.library.wur.nl/plcell/article/32/3/683/6099160

[95] Sakai K, Charlot F, Saux T Le, Bonhomme S, Nogué F, Palauqui JC, et al. Design of a comprehensive microfluidic and microscopic toolbox for the ultra-wide spatio-temporal study of plant protoplasts development and physiology. Plant Methods [Internet]. 2019 Dec 24 [cited 2021 Jun 17];15(1):1-12. Available from: https://plantmethods.biomedcentral.com/articles/10.1186/s13007-019-0459-z

[96] Busch W, Moore BT, Martsberger B, Mace DL, Twigg RW, Jung J, et al. A microfluidic device and computational platform for high-throughput live imaging of gene expression. Nat Methods 2012 911 [Internet]. 2012 Sep 30 [cited 2021 Aug 4];9(11):1101-6. Available from: https://www.nature.com/articles/nmeth.2185

[97] Horowitz LF, Rodriguez AD, Ray T, Folch A. Microfluidics for interrogating live intact tissues [Internet]. Vol. 6, Microsystems and Nanoengineering. Springer Nature; 2020 [cited 2021 Jun 17]. p. 1-27. Available from: www.nature.com/micronano

[98] Cove DJ, Schild A, Ashton NW, Hartmann E. GENETIC AND PHYSIOLOGICAL STUDIES OF THE EFFECT OF LIGHT ON THE DEVELOPMENT OF THE MOSS, *PHYSCOMITRELLA PATENS*. Photochem Photobiol [Internet]. 1978 Feb 1 [cited 2021 Aug 24];27(2):249-54. Available from: https://onlinelibrary.wiley.com/doi/full/10.1111/j.1751-1097.1978.tb07596.x

[99] Kamisugi Y, Stackelberg M Von, Lang D, Care M, Reski R, Rensing SA, et al. A sequence-anchored genetic linkage map for the moss, *Physcomitrella patens*. Plant J [Internet]. 2008 Dec 1 [cited 2021 Sep 1];56(5):855-66. Available from: https://onlinelibrary.wiley.com/doi/full/10.1111/j.1365-313X.2008.03637.x

[100] Ding X, Pervere LM, Jr. CB, Bibeau JP, Khurana S, Butt AM, et al. Conditional genetic screen in *Physcomitrella patens* reveals a novel microtubule depolymerizing-end-tracking protein. PLOS Genet [Internet]. 2018 May 1 [cited 2021 Aug 24];14(5):e1007221. Available from:

https://journals.plos.org/plosgenetics/article?id=10.1371/journal.pgen.1007221

[101] Mohanasundaram B, Rajmane VB, Jogdand S V., Bhide AJ, Banerjee AK. Agrobacterium-mediated Tnt1 mutagenesis of moss protonemal filaments and generation of stable mutants with impaired gametophyte. Mol Genet Genomics 2019 2943 [Internet]. 2019 Jan 28 [cited 2021 Aug 24];294(3):583-96. Available from: https://link.springer.com/article/10.1007/s00438-019-01532-4

[102] Nakaoka Y, Miki T, Fujioka R, Uehara R, Tomioka A, Obuse C, et al. An Inducible RNA Interference System in *Physcomitrella patens* Reveals a Dominant Role of Augmin in Phragmoplast Microtubule Generation. Plant Cell [Internet]. 2012 Aug 10 [cited 2021 Aug 24];24(4):1478-93. Available from: https://academic.oup.com/plcell/article/24/4/1478/6102364

[103] Kubo M, Imai A, Nishiyama T, Ishikawa M, Sato Y, Kurata T, et al. System for Stable β-Estradiol-Inducible Gene Expression in the Moss *Physcomitrella patens*. PLoS One [Internet]. 2013 Sep 27 [cited 2021 Aug 24];8(9):e77356. Available from: https://journals.plos.org/plosone/article?id=10.1371/journal.pone.0077356

[104] Bezanilla M, Perroud P-F, Pan A, Klueh P, Quatrano RS. An RNAi System in *Physcomitrella patens* with an Internal Marker for Silencing Allows for Rapid Identification of Loss of Function Phenotypes. Plant Biol [Internet]. 2005 Apr 15 [cited 2021 Aug 24];7(03):251-7. Available from: http://www.thieme-connect.com/products/ejournals/html/10.1055/s-2005-837597

[105] Bezanilla M. The Bezanilla Lab Moss Methods [Internet]. 2012 [cited 2021 Sep 2]. Available from: https://sites.dartmouth.edu/bezanillalab/moss-methods/

[106] Aoyama T, Hiwatashi Y, Shigyo M, Kofuji R, Kubo M, Ito M, et al. AP2-type transcription factors determine stem cell identity in the moss *Physcomitrella patens*. Development [Internet]. 2012 Sep 1 [cited 2021 Aug 20];139(17):3120-9. Available from: http://genome.jgi-psf.org/Phypa11/

[107] Ulfstedt M, Hu G-Z, Johansson M, Ronne H. Testing of Auxotrophic Selection Markers for Use in the Moss Physcomitrella Provides New Insights into the Mechanisms of Targeted Recombination. Front Plant Sci. 2017 Nov 3;0:1850.

[108] Lang D, Ullrich KK, Murat F, Fuchs J, Jenkins J, Haas FB, et al. The *Physcomitrella patens* chromosome-scale assembly reveals moss genome structure and evolution. Plant J [Internet]. 2018 Feb 1 [cited 2021 Aug 20];93(3):515-33. Available from: https://onlinelibrary.wiley.com/doi/full/10.1111/tpj.13801

[109] de Keijzer J, Kieft H, Ketelaar T, Goshima G, Janson ME. Shortening of Microtubule Overlap Regions Defines Membrane Delivery Sites during Plant Cytokinesis. Curr Biol. 2017 Feb 20;27(4):514-20.

[110] Lopez-Obando M, Hoffmann B, Géry C, Guyon-Debast A, Téoulé E, Rameau C, et al. Simple and Efficient Targeting of Multiple Genes Through CRISPR-Cas9 in *Physcomitrella patens*. G3 Genes|Genomes|Genetics [Internet]. 2016 Nov 1 [cited 2021 Aug 24];6(11):3647-53. Available from: https://academic.oup.com/g3journal/article/6/11/3647/6031123

[111] Mallett DR, Chang M, Cheng X, Bezanilla M. Efficient and modular CRISPR-Cas9 vector system for *Physcomitrella patens*. Plant Direct [Internet]. 2019 Sep 1 [cited 2021 Aug 24];3(9):e00168. Available from: https://onlinelibrary.wiley.com/doi/full/10.1002/pld3.168

[112] Concordet J-P, Haeussler M. CRISPOR: intuitive guide selection for CRISPR/Cas9 genome editing experiments and screens. Nucleic Acids Res [Internet]. 2018 Jul 2 [cited 2021 Sep 2];46(W1):W242-5. Available from: https://academic.oup.com/nar/article/46/W1/W242/4995687

[113] Yi P, Goshima G. Transient cotransformation of CRISPR/Cas9 and oligonucleotide templates enables efficient editing of target loci in *Physcomitrella patens*. Plant Biotechnol J [Internet]. 2020 Mar 1 [cited 2021 Aug 24];18(3):599-601. Available from: https://onlinelibrary.wiley.com/doi/full/10.1111/pbi.13238

[114] Vives C, Charlot F, Mhiri C, Contreras B, Daniel J, Epert A, et al. Highly efficient gene tagging in the bryophyte *Physcomitrella patens* using the tobacco (*Nicotiana tabacum*) Tnt1 retrotransposon. New Phytol [Internet]. 2016 Nov 1 [cited 2021 Aug 24];212(3):759-69. Available from: https://nph.onlinelibrary.wiley.com/doi/full/10.1111/nph.14152

[115] Roberts AW, Dimos CS, Budziszek MJ, Goss CA, Lai V. Knocking Out the Wall: Protocols for Gene Targeting in *Physcomitrella patens* BT - The Plant Cell Wall: Methods and Protocols. In: Popper ZA, editor. Totowa, NJ: Humana Press; 2011. p. 273-90. Available from: https://doi.org/10.1007/978-1-61779-008-9_19

[116] Schaefer DG. Gene targeting in *Physcomitrella patens*. Curr Opin Plant Biol. 2001 Apr 1;4(2):143-50.

[117] Hohe A, Egener T, Lucht JM, Holtorf H, Reinhard C, Schween G, et al. An improved and highly standardised transformation procedure allows efficient production of single and multiple targeted gene-knockouts in a moss, *Physcomitrella patens*. Curr Genet 2003 446 [Internet]. 2003 Oct 29 [cited 2021 Aug 24];44(6):339-47. Available from: https://link.springer.com/article/10.1007/s00294-003-0458-4

[118] Li LH, Yang J, Qiu HL, Liu YY. Genetic transformation of *Physcomitrella patens* mediated by *Agrobacterium tumefaciens*. African J Biotechnol. 2010;9(25):3719-25.

[119] Cho S-H, Chung Y-S, Cho S-K, Rim Y-W, Shin and J-S. Particle Bombardment Mediated Transformation and GFP Expression in the Moss *Physcomitrella patens*. Mol Cells [Internet]. 1999 [cited 2021 Aug 24];9(1):14-9. Available from: http://www.molcells.org/journal/view.html?spage=14&volume=9&number=1

[120] Prihatna C, Chen R, Barbetti MJ, Barker SJ, Tuset SI, Demirer GS, et al. Phyllotaxis: A Matthew Effect in Auxin Action Dolf. Adv Phytonanotechnology [Internet]. 2019 Mar 1 [cited 2020 Jan 30];1(1):1-12. Available from: http://dx.doi.org/10.1038/s42003-020-0917-1

[121] Nomura T, Sakurai T, Osakabe Y, Osakabe K, Sakakibara H. Efficient and Heritable Targeted Mutagenesis in Mosses Using the CRISPR/Cas9 System. Plant Cell Physiol [Internet]. 2016 Dec 1 [cited 2021 Sep 7];57(12):2600-10. Available from: https://academic.oup.com/pcp/article/57/12/2600/2629317

[122] Kirbis A, Waller M, Ricca M, Bont Z, Neubauer A, Goffinet B, et al. Transcriptional Landscapes of Divergent Sporophyte Development in Two Mosses, Physcomitrium (Physcomitrella) patens and *Funaria hygrometrica*. Front Plant Sci. 2020 Jun 10;0:747.

[123] Mao L, Kawaide H, Higuchi T, Chen M, Miyamoto K, Hirata Y, et al. Genomic evidence for convergent evolution of gene clusters for momilactone biosynthesis in land plants. Proc Natl Acad Sci [Internet]. 2020 Jun 2 [cited 2021 Sep 7];117(22):12472-80. Available from:

https://www-pnas-org.ezproxy.library.wur.nl/content/117/22/12472

[124] Weston DJ, Turetsky MR, Johnson MG, Granath G, Lindo Z, Belyea LR, et al. The Sphagnome Project: enabling ecological and evolutionary insights through a genus-level sequencing project. New Phytol [Internet]. 2018 Jan 1 [cited 2021 Sep 7];217(1):16-25. Available from: https://nph.onlinelibrary.wiley.com/doi/full/10.1111/nph.14860

[125] Yu J, Li L, Wang S, Dong S, Chen Z, Patel N, et al. Draft genome of the aquatic moss *Fontinalis antipyretica* (Fontinalaceae, Bryophyta). Gigabyte [Internet]. 2020 Nov 16 [cited 2021 Sep 7];2020:1-9. Available from: https://gigabytejournal.com/articles/8

[126] Silva AT, Gao B, Fisher KM, Mishler BD, Ekwealor JTB, Stark LR, et al. To dry perchance to live: Insights from the genome of the desiccation-tolerant biocrust moss *Syntrichia caninervis*. Plant J [Internet]. 2021 Mar 1 [cited 2021 Sep 7];105(5):1339-56. Available from: https://onlinelibrary-wiley-com.ezproxy.library.wur.nl/doi/full/10.1111/tpj.15116

[127] Carey SB, Jenkins J, Lovell JT, Maumus F, Sreedasyam A, Payton AC, et al. Gene-rich UV sex chromosomes harbor conserved regulators of sexual development. Sci Adv. 2021 Jun 1;7(27).

[128] Horn A, Pascal A, Lončarević I, Marques RV, Lu Y, Miguel S, et al. Natural Products from Bryophytes: From Basic Biology to Biotechnological Applications. https://doi-org.ezproxy.library.wur.nl/101080/0735268920211911034 [Internet]. 2021 [cited 2021 Sep 7];40(3):191-217. Available from: https://www-tandfonline-com.ezproxy.library.wur.nl/doi/abs/10.1080/07352689.2021.1911034

[129] Campos ML, Prado GS, dos Santos VO, Nascimento LC, Dohms SM, da Cunha NB, et al. Mosses: Versatile plants for biotechnological applications. Vol. 41, Biotechnology Advances. Elsevier Inc.; 2020. p. 107533.

[130] Biersma EM, Convey P, Wyber R, Robinson SA, Dowton M, van de Vijver B, et al. Latitudinal Biogeographic Structuring in the Globally Distributed Moss *Ceratodon purpureus*. Front Plant Sci. 2020 Aug 28;0:1332.

[131] Kollar LM, Kiel S, James AJ, Carnley CT, Scola DN, Clark TN, et al. The genetic architecture of sexual dimorphism in the moss *Ceratodon purpureus*. Proc R Soc B [Internet]. 2021 Mar 10 [cited 2021 Sep 8];288(1946). Available from: https://royalsocietypublishing-org.ezproxy.library.wur.nl/doi/abs/10.1098/rspb.2020.2908

[132] Slate ML, Rosenstiel TN, Eppley SM. Sex-specific morphological and physiological differences in the moss *Ceratodon purpureus* (Dicranales). Ann Bot [Internet]. 2017 Nov 10 [cited 2021 Sep 8];120(5):845-54. Available from: https://academic.oup.com/aob/article/120/5/845/3947929

[133] Trouiller B, Charlot F, Choinard S, Schaefer DG, Nogué F. Comparison of gene targeting efficiencies in two mosses suggests that it is a conserved feature of Bryophyte transformation. Biotechnol Lett 2007 2910 [Internet]. 2007 Jun 13 [cited 2021 Sep 8];29(10):1591-8. Available from: https://link.springer.com/article/10.1007/s10529-007-9423-5

[134] Pederson ERA, Warshan D, Rasmussen U. Genome Sequencing of *Pleurozium schreberi*: The Assembled and Annotated Draft Genome of a Pleurocarpous Feather Moss. G3 Genes, Genomes, Genet [Internet]. 2019 Sep 1 [cited 2021 Sep 7];9(9):2791-7. Available from: https://www.g3journal.org/content/9/9/2791

[135] Heck MA, Lüth VM, Gessel N van, Krebs M, Kohl M, Prager A, et al. Axenic in vitro cultivation of 19 peat moss (Sphagnum L.) species as a resource for basic biology, biotechnology, and paludiculture. New Phytol [Internet]. 2021 Jan 1 [cited 2021 Sep 8];229(2):861-76. Available from: https://nph-onlinelibrary-wiley-com.ezproxy.library.wur.nl/doi/full/10.1111/nph.16922

[136] Kariyawasam IU, Price MJ, Bell NE, Long DG, Mill RR, Hyvönen J. Unearthing a lectotype for *Polytrichum commune* Hedw. (Bryophyta, Polytrichaceae). Taxon [Internet]. 2021 Jun 1 [cited 2021 Sep 7];70(3):653-9. Available from: https://onlinelibrary.wiley.com/doi/full/10.1002/tax.12444

[137] Goryunov D V., Sotnikova EA, Goryunova S V., Kuznetsova OI, Logacheva MD, Milyutina IA, et al. The Mitochondrial Genome of Nematodontous Moss *Polytrichum commune* and Analysis of Intergenic Repeats Distribution Among Bryophyta. Divers 2021, Vol 13, Page 54 [Internet]. 2021 Feb 1 [cited 2021 Sep 6];13(2):54. Available from: https://www.mdpi.com/1424-2818/13/2/54/htm

[138] Jin X-J, Zhu R-L. The complete plastome of *Polytrichum commune* Hedw. (Polytrichaceae, Bryophyta). http://www-tandfonline-com.ezproxy.library.wur.nl/action/authorSubmission?journalCode=tmdn20&page=instructions [Internet]. 2021 [cited 2021 Sep 7];6(5):1645-7. Available from: https://www-tandfonline-com.ezproxy.library.wur.nl/doi/abs/10.1080/23802359.2021.1927223

[139] Pan Z, Pitt WG, Zhang Y, Wu N, Tao Y, Truscott TT. The upside-down water collection system of *Syntrichia caninervis*. Nat Plants 2016 27 [Internet]. 2016 Jun 6 [cited 2021 Sep 8];2(7):1-5. Available from: https://www.nature.com/articles/nplants201676

[140] Rahmatpour N, Perera N V., Singh V, Wegrzyn JL, Goffinet B. High gene space divergence contrasts with frozen vegetative architecture in the moss family Funariaceae. Mol Phylogenet Evol. 2021 Jan 1;154:106965.

Section 3

Model Crops and Trait Improvement

Chapter 4

Maize (*Zea mays* L.) as a Model System for Plant Genetic, Genomic, and Applied Research

Fakhriddin N. Kushanov, Ozod S. Turaev,
Oybek A. Muhammadiyev, Ramziddin F. Umarov,
Nargiza M. Rakhimova and Noilabonu N. Mamadaliyeva

Abstract

Maize leads the world's cereals after wheat and rice in terms of cultivated area, because of its economic importance for the production of both food purposes and raw materials for industry. The maize genus *Zea* L. belonging to the family of cereals (*Poaceae* or *Graminaceae*) includes six species. However, all cultivated maize belongs specifically to *Zea mays* L. subsp. *mays* ($2n = 2\times = 20$) is the only cultivated species of the genus *Zea* L., and the remaining species of this genus are mostly wild herbaceous plants. In addition to meeting the nutritional needs of the world's population, *Zea mays* L. is one of the classic model objects of genetic and physiological research, as well as in the field of breeding not only cereals but also other important agricultural plants. Especially, this model object has been used in genetic mapping of loci of quantitative traits and genes associated with economically valuable traits, such as yield, resistance to diseases and pests, grain quality, etc. in cereal crops.

Keywords: *Zea mays* L., hybridization, cytoplasmic male sterility, QTL, mapping, GWAS

1. Introduction

Due to the constant growth of the world's population, the demand for high-calorie foods is increasing. Although maize was developed as an American crop, it is now grown all over the world and today it has become the third most important food crop after wheat and rice [1, 2]. Maize is the world's leading cereal after wheat and rice in terms of sown area, as currently makes up about 21% of the human diet worldwide and more than 500 different staples and additives are produced from it (FAOSTAT data). According to the International Grains Council (IGC), the corn grain harvest in 2021 was about 1.12 billion tons.

A special role in the genetic analysis is played by model objects, by working with which the researcher can significantly speed up and facilitate the process of analysis. Maize (*Zea mays* L.) is one of the main classical models for fundamental research in the fields of plant genetics and breeding. Especially, this model object has been used in genetic mapping of loci of quantitative traits and genes associated with economically valuable traits, such as yield, resistance to diseases and pests, grain quality, etc. in cereal crops. Since its chromosomes are easily analyzed under an optical microscope, maize is also suitable for plant cytogenetic analysis. The simplicity of castration (removal of male inflorescences—panicle), the presence of mutations that cause male sterility, the possibility of setting seeds both during cross-pollination and during self-pollination, the presence of a huge number of various mutations facilitates hybridization.

The genus *Zea* L. from the grass family (*Poaceae* or *Graminaceae*) is represented by four diploid (2n = 2× = 20) and one tetraploid (2n = 4× = 40) species;

1. *Zea diploperennis*—diploperennial teosinte,
2. *Zea luxurians*—teosinte,
3. *Zea nicaraguensis*,
4. *Zea mays* L.—corn are diploids, and
5. *Zea perennis*—perennial teosinte is a tetraploid species.

In turn, *Zea mays* L. is divided into three subspecies, such as,

1. *Zea mays* subsp. *huehuetenangensis*—maize,
2. *Zea mays* L. subsp. *mays* and
3. *Zea mays* subsp. *parviglumis*.

As well as there are three subspecies including

1. *Zea mays* subsp. *mays*—corn,
2. *Zea mays* subsp. *mexicana* (Schrad.), and
3. *Zea mays* subsp. *parviglumis*.

All species belonging to the genus *Zea* L. cross with other maize diploid species, except the perennial tetraploid *Z. perennis*. While, the diploid maize and its wild relative, teosinte *Zea perennis* (Hitchc.) Reeves & Mangelsd, readily intercrossing [3].

Maize (*Zea mays* L. subsp. *mays*) is the single cultivated species of the genus *Zea* L. The genome size of the diploid maize species ranges from 2.2 to 2.7 GB, including approximately 32.000–42.000 protein-coding genes [4, 5]. The first tetraploid species of *Zea mays* L. was obtained by Randolph (1932), using the heat shock method [6]. The tetraploid species is characterized by the strong development of all plant organs, resistance to abiotic and biotic environmental factors, and increased content of nutrients compared to diploid species [7].

Currently, genetic, chromosomal, genomic, and cytoplasmic modifications have been identified in maize, in particular, gene mutations have been best studied [4, 8, 9]. Especially, the genes that control the behavior of chromosomes in mitosis and meiosis, enzyme systems, the formation of chlorophyll and other pigments have been studied and described; structures and functions of vegetative organs, structure, and color of the endosperm, regulatory systems responsible for the mutability and expression of other genes, for the development of various elements of the reproductive system, which determine male and female sterility, selective fertilization, etc. [4, 8, 10].

Moreover, in maize were found and well-studied spontaneous and induced chromosome rearrangements such as deficiencies, translocations, duplications, and inversions [4]. In recent years, translocations have been widely used in maize to determine linkage groups [8].

Since the discovery of polyploidy forms of maize, many of them have been well studied. They are found in the aneuploids—trisomics, and monosomics in maize [8]. On maize, cytological evidence of crossing over was obtained for the first time in plants and mobile genetic elements were discovered [8, 11]. It studied the influence of long-term inbreeding and the effects of heterosis in plants and developed hybrid breeding techniques based on obtaining and crossing pure lines (interline and double interline hybrids); cytoplasmic mutations are well studied, especially mutations associated with cytoplasmic male sterility (CMS), the use of which is one of the achievements of maize genetics and plant genetics in general.

2. The origin and evolution of maize

Even though the origin of maize has been studied in-depth, it remains controversial. Prehistoric breeder practitioners who cannot live and reproduce in their current form without human help [12] domesticated maize (*Zea mays* L.). After the American continent was discovered, it became clear that corn was the staple food of the endemic Indians on the continent. According to several authors, maize was introduced into cultivation 7–12.000 years ago in the territory of southwestern Mexico. Cave excavations in arid regions of Mexico have unearthed small grains of corn grown for food 5.000 years ago [13]. The oldest finds of cultivated corn kernels were discovered in the caves of Gwila Nakitz and Tehuacan, located in the northwestern state of Oaxaca and the southeastern state of Puebla in central Mexico. In addition, according to archaeobotanists Ranere et al. (2009), the first straight there is evidence that maize was domesticated about 8.700 years ago in the Balsas region from the wild teosinte plant [14].

Taxonomic and evolutionary studies indicate that the teosinte is the closest wild relative of four annual and perennial maize species of the genus *Zea* L. [3]. However, according to the authors, some species of teosinte are genetically and taxonomically differing from *Zea mays* L. While, in the study of maize genetics, researchers consider *teosinte* to be an important resource.

Thus, according to archaeobotanical findings and the results of traditional analyzes [12, 13], there are various theories about the origin of *Zea mays* L. ssp. mays:

1. As a result of the selection of the wild subspecies *Zea mays* ssp. *parviglumis*. In addition, due to the possible introgressive hybridization with the ancestral form *Z. mays* ssp. *mexicana*, the genetic material of up to 12% of cultivated form might be obtained from this subspecies.

2. Caused by the hybridization of small cultivated wild form with another species of this genus—either *Z. luxurians* or *Z. diploperennis*.

3. One wild form has been introduced into the crop several times.

4. From the hybridization of *Zea diploperennis* with some representatives of the closely related genus *Tripsacum*.

3. Maize polyploidy studies

Polyploidy or whole-genome duplication (WGD) is considered as a major process in plant evolution. A polyploidy event 160 million years ago is theorized to have created the ancestral line that led to all modern flowering plants [15]. Genome duplication is categorized into two events paleopolyploidy (ancient polyploidy) and neopolyploidy (recent polyploidy). Ancient genome duplications are widespread throughout eukaryotic lineages, particularly in plants. Paleopolyploidy has occurred at least several million years ago. Both phenomena, ancient and recent polyploids could occur through the doubling of the genome of single species (autopolyploidy) or combining genomes of two different species (allopolyploidy).

According to the maize DNA sequence data, the genome duplications event occurred after the divergence between sorghum and maize [10]. The duplications event that happened approximately 11.4 million years ago resulted from an ancient polyploid [16]. The maize WGD resulted in the subgenomes maize1 and maize2 [17]. Polyploids are found almost in all groups of eukaryotic organisms as a result of incorrect meiosis, fertilization, or cell division [18]. Polyploids can be obtained experimentally by treatment with chemicals such as colchicine, oryzalin, trifluralin and amiprophosmethyl or by combining diploid nuclei.

Niazi et al. (2014) have studied induced polyploidy in maize hybrids to increase heterosis and restore reproductive fertility [19]. The seeds of open-pollinated maize breeding lines and a maize × teosinte cross were germinated in colchicine solution (0.25, 0.5, or 1.0%) until they had a thick radical and protruded plumule. The highest number of tetraploids with the lowest number of chimeric plants induced at 0.5% colchicine. Scientists have reported that the leaf area, total soluble solids, leaf oil percentage, and leaf crude protein contents were significantly increased in leaves of the induced tetraploids of maize and maize × teosinte crosses relative to the diploid subspecies.

Iqbal et al. (2018) have conducted research aimed to clarify the mysterious meiotic behavior of autopolyploid and allopolyploid maize [20]. Scientists have explored the stability of the chromosomes during meiosis in both auto- and allopolyploid maize. Furthermore, they have identified an association of chromosomes between maize and *Z. perennis* by obtaining a numerous of auto- and allopolyploid maize hybrids. The results showed a higher level of chromosome stability in allopolyploid maize during meiosis than in autopolyploid maize. Additionally, the meiotic behavior of *Z. perennis* was relatively more stable than the allopolyploid maize. As well as, 10 chromosomes of maize "A" subgenomes were homologous to 20 chromosomes of *Z. perennis* genome with little evolutionary differentiation and a higher pairing frequency. However, "A" subgenome chromosomes have shown a little evolutionary differentiation, while "B" subgenome chromosomes had a lower pairing frequency and higher evolutionary differentiation in maize.

The diversity analysis of wild relatives of maize showed that various genes have different histories and domestication such as intensive breeding processes have had heterogeneous effects on genetic diversity across genes [10].

4. Maize is a model in genetic mapping studies for cereal crop improvement

4.1 QTL mapping and GWAS for dissecting genetic architecture of complex traits

A quantitative trait is a measurable phenotype and varies continuously among individuals in a population. Quantitative trait loci (QTL) are genomic regions in which genetic segregation within a population is statistically associated with variation in a quantitative trait. Genetic mapping of QTL is a process of locating genes with effects on quantitative traits using molecular markers. QTL mapping is a powerful method for improving agricultural crops, which allows using marker-assisted selection technology to introgression the genes of interest from one genotype to another [21].

QTL mapping and genome-wide association study (GWAS) both are similar and they typically measure the associations between genotype and phenotype [21, 22]. GWAS is a powerful tool for dissecting the genetic architecture of complex traits in many crop species [22–24]. The main goal of GWAS is to link genotypic variations with phenotypic differences. With the development of whole-genome sequencing technology and high-density single-nucleotide polymorphism (SNP) BeadCap, GWAS has also begun to be widely used to identify candidate genes that control quantitative traits in crops [22].

Maize is a suitable crop for the GWAS approach and considerable progress has been made over the last decade [25]. GWAS has been successfully used in maize to detect a great many candidate QTL/genes attending to control diverse morpho-biological and economically important traits, such as salt [26–28] and drought tolerance [8, 23, 29–31], kernel traits [32–36] and many other traits of interest. GWAS facilitates to achieve advances in current studies in quantitative genetics.

4.2 Genetic analysis and fine mapping of QTL for kernel traits

Grain traits are the most important in maize commercialization over the world. Kernel sizes and weight are major traits for grain yield in maize. Liu et al. (2014) was conducted the genetic analysis and identified major QTL for maize kernel size and weight [37]. They have identified a total of 55 and 28 QTL of maize kernel-size traits and kernel weight using composite interval mapping (CIM) for single-environment analysis along with mixed linear model-based CIM for joint analysis, respectively.

Wang et al. (2020) have conducted QTL analysis and fine mapping using a composite interval mapping (CIM) method aimed to map QTLs and predict candidate genes for kernel size in maize [38]. Five QTL were identified for kernel length and five QTL for kernel width out of 10 QTL.

Pan et al. (2017) reported the results of QTL mapping in six environments and consensus loci for grain weight detected by meta-analysis [39]. Subsequently, a meta-analysis was performed and 62 QTLs were determined for grain weight, ear weight, and kernel weight per plant in six environments.

Li et al. (2010) have carried out QTL mapping for grain yield and yield components under high and low phosphorus treatments in maize [40]. 69 QTL were identified for the six traits at two sites. Thirty-six distinct QTL were identified from Taian, in which 7 out of 36 for grain yield, 7 for 100 kernel weight, 5 for ear length, 5 for per ear, 6 for kernel number per row, and 6 for ear diameter, while 33 distinct QTLs were identified at Yantai, in which 6 out of 33 for grain yield, 5 for 100 kernel weight, 5 for ear length, 7 for row number per ear, 5 for kernel number per row and 5 for ear diameter.

Liu et al. (2020) have identification of QTL for kernel-related traits and the heterosis for these traits [34]. They developed and evaluated 301 RILs population for six kernel-related traits and the mid-parent heterosis (MPH) for these traits. A total of 100 QTLs were identified in both mapping populations. As well, 20 QTL clusters including 46 QTLs were identified across ten chromosomes. These results may provide additional insights into the genetic basis for the mid-parent heterosis for kernel-related traits.

Liu et al. (2015) conducted a genetic analysis of kernel traits in maize-teosinte introgression populations [33]. Scientists have analyzed kernel morphological traits in 10 maize-teosinte introgression populations using digital imaging software. QTLs were identified for kernel area and length with moderate allelic effects that colocalize with kernel weight QTL.

Another group of researchers has conducted linkage and association mapping aims to the analysis of the genetic architecture of maize kernel size [34]. Three kernel traits of maize, kernel length, kernel width, and kernel thickness, were studied in germplasm accessions and a biparental population. A total of 21 SNPs were identified under four environments. Besides, 50 QTL were determined in seven environments doubled haploid population. Combining the two mapping populations revealed that 56 SNPs fell within 18 of the QTL confidence intervals. A total of 73 candidate genes were detected, regulating seed development. As well, seven miRNAs were found to locate within the linkage disequilibrium regions of the colocalized SNPs.

Jiang et al. (2013) performed a meta-analysis of 584 QTLs related to grain yield components [41]. A total of 73 Meta-QTLs for grain yield components such as 22 QTLs for row number, 7 QTLs for kernel number per row, and 44 QTLs for kernel weight were estimated. Another group of Chinese scientists carried out combining meta-QTL with RNA-seq data to identify candidate genes of kernel row number traits [42]. A total of 373 QTL for grain yield and kernel row number was meta-analyzed. Fifty-four meta-QTL were determined, including 19 for grain yield and 35 for kernel row number. A total of 1.588 genes located in the kernel row number meta-QTL regions were identified by gene expression data.

DNA markers associated with kernel traits could be applied to marker-assisted selection (MAS) to facilitate yield architecture, QTL fine mapping, and gene cloning in the maize community [42].

4.3 The maize multiparental populations advance mapping resolution and power

4.3.1 Maize-NAM population as a template for other crops

Molecular mapping is typically carried out using genetically segregated F_2, backcross (BC), recombinant inbred lines (RIL), doubled haploids (DH), and near-isogenic lines (NIL). These commonly used biparental populations have their weaknesses such as lower power, limited recombination, temporary nature, the impossibility of estimation of dominant effects, time requirement, and expense. To overcome some of the shortcomings in quantitative trait locus (QTL) mapping in biparental populations, schemes for creating mapping populations with multiple parental genotypes have been developed. The genetic diversity of these types of populations along with causing a wide range of phenotypes, it makes possible to identify QTLs with high accuracy.

The nested association mapping (NAM) population is also an example of the experimental design for multiparental populations (**Figure 1**). The NAM strategy was first developed in collaboration with researchers Buckler et al. [43] to study the genetic architecture of complex traits of maize (*Zea mays* L.). It should be noted that, unlike association mapping, NAM is a unique method that is performed only in a specially developed population [43].

The theory of nested association mapping

The main goal of the NAM is to efficiently link phenotypic traits with genotypic data, as in a traditional QTL mapping strategy. The NAM method with low marker

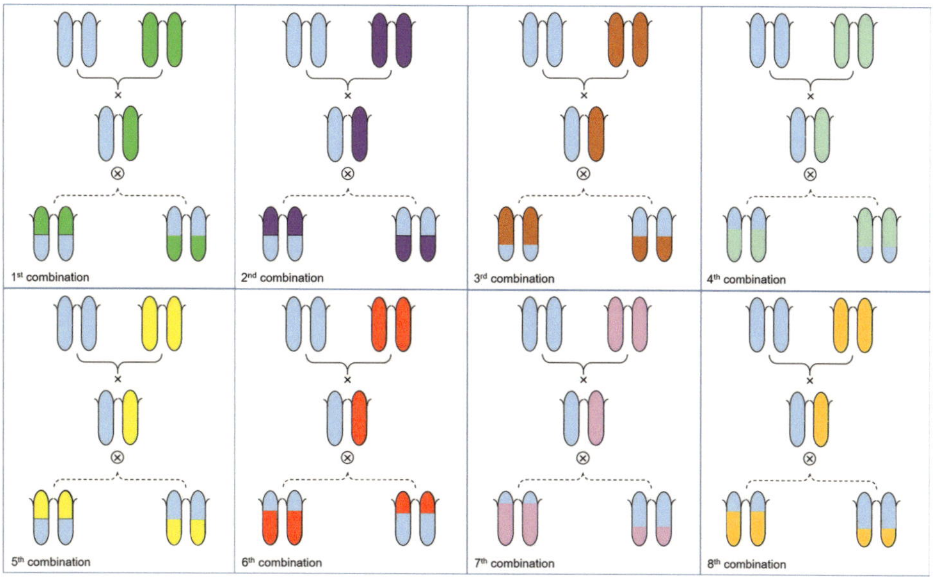

Figure 1.
The nested association mapping (NAM) population scheme.

density, high allele richness, high mapping resolution, and high statistical power overcomes the disadvantages of Linkage analysis and Association mapping as well took advantages of both methods.

The NAM strategy allows researchers to effectively apply systematic methods of genetics and genomics and create sources such as general mapping populations as well to explore complex traits of plants at the fundamental level.

The NAM strategy involves the following stages [43]:

1. Selection of diverse founders and the development of a mapping population (RILs with a stable set of phenotypic traits are preferred);

2. Sequencing or high-density genotyping of parental genotypes;

3. Genotyping of both the founders and the progenies with a smaller number of tagging markers to explain the inheritance of chromosome segments and to project the high-density marker information from the founders to the progenies;

4. Phenotyping of hybrids/RILs for various complex traits;

5. Conducting genome-wide association analysis using genotypic and phenotypic data.

The maize-NAM population was developed by crossing 25 diverse founders to a single common inbred line, B73, resulting in 5.000 RILs. Buckler et al. (2009) reported the results of the study on the genetic architecture of flowering time using the maize-NAM population [44, 45]. Subsequently, several NAM populations in maize were developed such as in Dent and Flint maize [46], Chinese inbred lines population-based NAM [47], and teosinte [48].

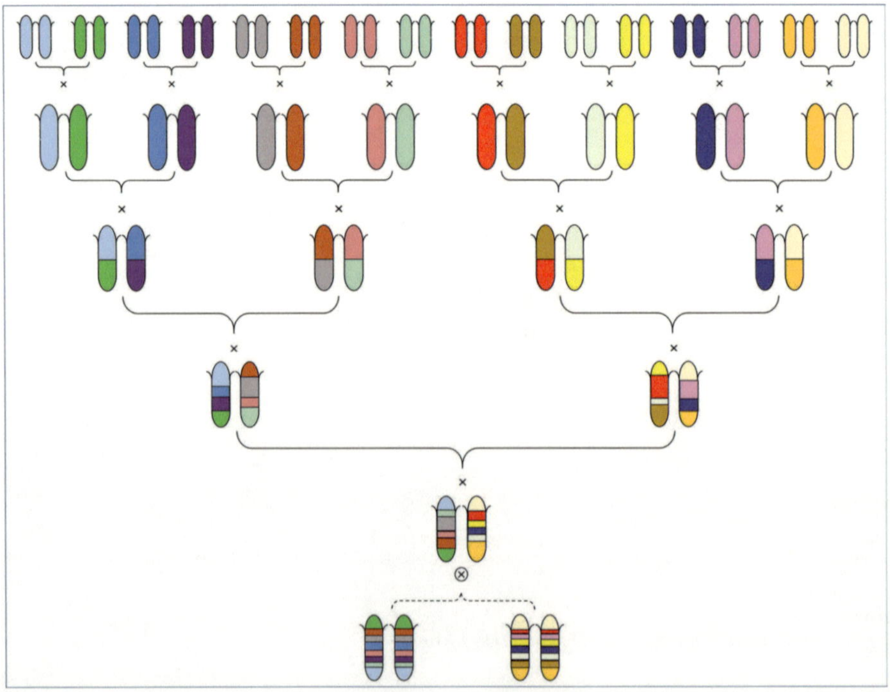

Figure 2.
Multi-parent advanced generation inter-cross (MAGIC) population scheme.

The maize-NAM design served as a model for other crops such as sorghum [1, 49–51], peanut [52, 53], barley [11, 54–57], oilseed rape [22, 58], wheat [59–63], rice [64, 65], soybean [66, 67] and cotton [68, 69] as well as NAM were developed in the model plant *Arabidopsis thaliana* [70, 71].

4.3.2 MAGIC population with greatly reduce mating design

Over the past decade, the use of multiparental populations was increased in plant genetic research. The two most popular multiparental population designs in crops are NAM and MAGIC (multi-parent advanced generation inter-cross) populations (**Figure 2**) [72]. MAGIC populations offer new opportunities in genetic mapping strategies and crop breeding approaches due to their complex pedigree structure [73]. MAGIC was first proposed and applied in mice [74], as well as Mackay and Powell (2007), and Cavanagh et al. (2008) first discussed in plants [75, 76]. The first plant-MAGIC population was developed in *A. thaliana* parents [77].

According to the MAGIC designs [75], several inbred lines are intercrossed many times over in aiming to assemble mosaic parental alleles in a single line (**Figure 1**). Two different MAGIC populations were developed in maize [78–80].

Dell'Acqua et al. (2015) produced 1.636 MAGIC maize RILs derived from eight genetically diverse inbred lines [79]. They show how MAGIC maize may find strong candidate genes by incorporating genome sequencing and transcriptomics data. They discuss several QTL for grain yield and flowering time, reporting candidate genes. Anderson et al. (2018) were developed four parent maize populations with five different mating designs used in MAGIC and bi-parental populations including 1.149 individuals [78]. The combined population here is comprised of 118.509 genetic markers. They conducted association mapping and identified 2, 5, 7, and 6 QTL for plant height, ear height, days to anthesis, and silking, respectively [78].

5. "Omics" tools to understand molecular mechanisms of major traits

5.1 RNAi and genome editing tools for control gene expression

The possibility of using an organism's own gene and systematically inducing and triggering RNA interference (RNAi) for any desired sequence made RNAi an effective approach for functional genomics [81]. RNAi is a major biological process in plants that causes gene silencing both transcriptionally and post-transcriptionally. RNAi has been widely used in crops since its discovery. To date, this approach has been conventionally based on the use of transgenic plants expressing double-stranded RNAs (dsRNAs) against selected targets [82].

Segal et al. (2003) have conducted initial studies on RNAi mechanisms in maize [83]. They found that maize transformed RNAi constructs for 22-kD zein gene suppression could produce a dominant opaque phenotype. This phenotype suppresses 22-kD zeins without affecting the accumulation of other zein proteins.

Casati et al. (2006) have conducted GWAS of high-altitude maize and gene knockdown stocks implicate chromatin-remodeling proteins in response to UV-B [84]. They implemented comparative analysis by expression profiling of maize aim to determine new components in the mechanisms of maize responses to UV-B. Microarray analysis illustrated that among the UV-B responsive transcripts, various types of genes implicated in chromatin remodeling are differentially expressed before and after UV-B treatment in high-altitude lines. Transgenic RNAi plants with lower expression of four chromatin-associated genes showed hypersensitivity to UV-B, and altered UV-B regulation of selected genes. The results showed that genes attended in chromatin remodeling are crucial for UV-B acclimation and that some lines illustrate adaptations to this challenge.

Besides, Casati and Walbot (2008) have reported different transcriptome changes in RNAi lines. They used 44 K Agilent oligonucleotide array platform to compare RNAi lines to each other and to UV-B tolerant nontransgenic siblings both before and after 8 h of UV-B exposure [85]. Maize leaves express more than 20.000 different transcripts under greenhouse conditions; after UV-B exposure 267 transcripts exhibit expression changes in control genotypes of B73.

In recent years, RNAi research in maize has been developing rapidly. One of the agricultural economic problem is aflatoxins that are produced by fungus species such as *Aspergillus*. In spite of control efforts, aflatoxin contamination is causing the global loss of crops productions each year. Thakare et al. (2017) have obtained aflatoxin-free transgenic maize using host-induced gene silencing [86]. Scientists show that host-induced gene silencing is an effective method for eliminating this toxin in transgenic maize. They transformed RNAi-gene cassette targeting *aflC* gene, which encodes an enzyme in the Aspergillus aflatoxin biosynthetic pathway to the maize plants. The aflatoxin was not be detected in kernels of RNAi-maize plants after pathogen infection, while toxin loads reached thousands of parts per billion in nontransgenic control kernels. The results show that siRNA molecules can be used to silence aflatoxin biosynthesis in maize.

Velez et al. (2020) have studied the lethal and sublethal effects of Sec23 dsRNA in maize RNAi lines to control western corn rootworm (WCR) [87]. They determined Sec23 as a highly lethal RNAi target using WCR adult feeding assays. Scientists explain Sec23 dsRNA as an RNAi target for planta rootworm control.

In the last few years, new genome editing methods have emerged that use four types of engineered nucleases: Meganucleases, ZFN (Zinc-Finger Nucleases), TALENs (Transcription Activator Like Effector Nucleases), and the CRISPR (Clustered Regularly Interspaced Short Palindromic Repeats) system. Among model plants, including maize, all kinds of nucleases mentioned above have been used to create targeted genome modifications [88, 89]. For example, D'Halluin et al. (2008) reported the first use of targeted genome modification using customizable endonucleases in maize. They succeeded in inserting a 35S promoter upstream of a promoterless herbicide resistance transgene using a meganuclease [90]. Later, Shukla et al. (2009) reported the first use of ZFNs for site-directed mutagenesis at the maize *IPK1* gene as well as site-directed DNA insertion of a PAT gene [91]. Especially, among the DNA-Free Genome Editing technologies TALEN and CRISPR/cas9 technologies, have become powerful tools for genomic research. For the first time in maize, a group of scientists [92] using both TALEN and CRISPR systems reported the results of site-directed mutagenesis in maize. They designed 5 TALEN and two CRISPR constructions that target three genes involved in phytic acid (PA) biosynthesis. The results of this study served to reduce the content of PA in the seed and this led the authors to conclude that both technologies can be used to modify the maize genome. The following year, using this technology has been obtained the generation of stable, heritable mutations at the maize *glossy2* locus [93]. As a result of this study, transgenic plants containing mono- or diallelic mutations were obtained with a frequency of about 10%. However, the TALEN method is more labor-intensive, requiring more time for construction than CRISPR/Cas9.

Thus, the development of the TALEN and CRISPR/Cas9 systems is an important step in the development of modern genomic engineering. The emergence of these systems, due to their low cost and ease of design, has become a powerful impetus for the development of both fundamental and applied science. More precisely, directional editing of plant genomes can be used to solve both; the study of gene functions and obtain plants with new properties, such as resistance to pathogens, herbicides, metabolism changes, yield indicators, etc. [94].

5.2 Maize proteomics opens the way for an insight into the biology of cereal crop

In the natural conditions of growth or cultivation of a species, plants in the process of their growth and development are often affected by adverse environmental factors [95]. Under the influence of unfavorable conditions, the decrease in physiological processes and functions can reach critical levels that do not ensure the implementation of the genetic program of ontogenesis, energy metabolism, regulatory systems, protein metabolism, and other vital functions of the plant organism are disrupted [96].

The main feature of protein research at the end of the twentieth century is proteomics. Since proteomics complements the research of genomics, transcriptomics, and metabolomics, it plays a central role in systems biology. Over the past three decades, significant progress has been made in the proteomic studies of maize as a model object [97]. Maize proteomic studies can be divided into two categories [98]:

1. Profiling (or mapping) of the identified proteins of biological material, with the aim of separating, identifying, and cataloging as many proteins as possible, and, thus, the most complete scanning of the expressed genome sequences in individual representatives, at certain phases of development.

2. Functional (cell-mapped) proteomics—studies polymorphism between different protein populations. With the help of two-dimensional electrophoresis, a

comparative analysis of protein extracts of control and experimental plants is carried out. Both types of analysis became more real and informative after the sequencing of the reference genotype of maize B73 was completed [10, 98].

To date, published maize proteomic studies have used major proteomic technologies such as SDS-PAGE and two-dimensional electrophoresis (2-DE), laser capture microdissection, a combination of 2-DE with time-of-flight mass spectrometry (MALDI TOF), gas chromatography-mass spectrometry technologies [99–104]. The main proteomic studies served to study changes in the composition of proteins under the influence of biotic and abiotic factors. For example, the effect of salicylic acid under high-temperature stress on the growth of seedlings and the antioxidant defense system of corn was studied [105]. In addition, the effect of some phytohormones, such as salicylic acid (SA), abscisic acid (ABA), jasmonic acid (JA), and methyl jasmonate (MeJA), on the protein composition of corn roots and leaves has been studied, and their important role in plant defenses has been proven [7, 98, 101, 105, 106].

However, despite the potential role of proteomics in advancing the study of stress tolerance in plants (also in the model), little useful information has been obtained so far for crop improvement and breeding [99].

5.3 Maize is a paragon for investigation of epigenetic studies

Epigenetic gene regulation is essential for the proper development of organisms. Epigenetic changes such as DNA methylation, histone modification, and RNA processing influence gene expression without changing the DNA sequence. Epigenetic studies have been the focus of many questions in plant research over the last decade [107]. The maize genome is relatively large and complex that includes abundant repetitive sequences, which are regularly silenced by epigenetic changes, making it an ideal organism to study epigenetic gene regulation. The application of new technologies to characterize maize epigenomes allows an understanding of the relationship between epigenetic mechanisms and genome organization [108].

Initial examples of epigenetic regulation were related to the transposable elements, starting with McClintock's early work in the 1950s [109]. Implementation of advanced technologies to describe maize epigenomes allows a more clear understanding of the association between epigenetic mechanisms and genome organization. In maize, the genome-wide analysis of cytosine methylation was carried out using the combination of high-throughput DNA sequencing with the enzymatic characterization of methylated bases through bisulfite conversion. In recent years, numerous genome-wide studies of cytosine methylation have been published in maize [30, 80, 110–115].

Eichten et al. (2011) have studied heritable epigenetic variation among maize inbred lines [111]. The comparison analysis of the DNA methylation degree of B73 and Mo17 maize lines permitted determining of about 700 differentially methylated regions (DMRs). Some DMRs occur in genomic regions that are apparently identical by descent in B73 and Mo17 suggesting that they may be examples of pure epigenetic variation. The results of this study showed the naturally occurring epigenetic variation in maize, including a pure epigenetic variation that is not conditioned by genetic differences. The identified epigenetic variation may provide complex trait variation.

Regulski et al. (2013) present the genome-wide map of cytosine methylation for two maize inbred lines, B73 and Mo17 [116]. Results showed that CpG (65%) and CpHpG (50%) islands (where H = A, C, or T) are highest methylated in transposons while CpHpH methylated is likely guided by 24-nucleotide (nt), but not 21-nt, small interfering RNAs (siRNAs). Scientists concluded that CpG methylation in exons (8%) may deter insertion of Mutator transposon insertion, while CpHpG methylation at splice acceptor sites may inhibit RNA splicing. The methylation map developed in this study will be an invaluable resource for maize epigenetic studies.

West et al. (2014) have studied the genomic distribution of H3K9me2 and DNA methylation in a maize genome [117]. They have investigated H3K9me2 in seedling tissue for the maize inbred B73 and compared to patterns of these modifications observed in Arabidopsis thaliana. This study gives a clear view of the relationship between DNA methylation and H3K9me2 in the maize genome and how the distribution of these modifications is shaped by the interplay of genes and transposons.

Kravets and Sokolova (2020) have studied the relationship between epigenetic variability with different individual radiosensitivity and adaptive capacity [118]. The researchers found significant differences in chromosomal aberration yield and DNA methylation profile under control and UV-C exposure for seedlings of subpopulations that differed in germination time. These significant differences in the control seedlings of different germination terms show the effect of the DNA methylation profile on DNA damage by regular metabolic factors including reactive oxygen species or thermal vibrations. The results showed the importance of epigenetic factors in identifying the radio-resistance and adaptive capacity of organisms.

Han et al. (2021) have reported epigenetic links to inbreeding depression in maize [119]. Throughout the subsequent inbreeding between inbred lines, thousands of genomic regions across TPC (teosinte branched1/cycloidea/proliferating cell factor)-binding sites (TBS) are hypermethylated across the H3K9me2-mediated pathway. Thus, several hundred TCP-target genes attended in mitochondrion, chloroplast, and ribosome functions are down-regulated, causing decreased growth vigor. On the contrary, random mating can reverse corresponding hypermethylation sites and TCP-target gene expression, restoring growth vigor.

A sufficiently large and highly repetitive maize genome provides an excellent model for other crop genomes to study gene regulation.

6. Conclusion and future prospect

More recently, plants have not played an important role in various genetic research because of their large and complex plant genomes. The role of model objects in understanding the patterns of historical and individual development of organisms is exceptionally great. The choice of an object for experimental scientific research, as a rule, becomes a separate task that requires special attention. It is necessary to clearly understand the criteria that the object of study must meet in order not only to solve the scientific problem, but also in its own way to facilitate the direct setting of the experiment. Plant genetics, physiology, and biochemistry have developed along this path, and the formation of modern sections of the biology of individual development is proceeding along this path.

Gradual studies carried out on model objects such as Arabidopsis, tobacco, and rice, including corn, proved that plants could also play a key role in molecular genetic experiments. Currently, genetic, chromosomal, genomic, and cytoplasmic modifications have been identified in maize; in particular, gene mutations have been best studied. To date, *Zea mays* L. is widely used in scientific research of the plant world. Day after day, it becomes a real classical model in plant biology; it has unconditional advantages in solving many current issues of genetics and individual development of plants, including cereals. Nevertheless, world science is moving forward and posing tasks that are ever more complex for researchers, for which corn alone is not enough.

Author details

Fakhriddin N. Kushanov[1,2*], Ozod S. Turaev[1,2], Oybek A. Muhammadiyev[1], Ramziddin F. Umarov[1], Nargiza M. Rakhimova[1] and Noilabonu N. Mamadaliyeva[1]

1 Institute of Genetics and Plant Experimental Biology, Academy of Sciences of the Republic of Uzbekistan, Tashkent, Uzbekistan

2 Department of Biology, National University of Uzbekistan, Tashkent, Uzbekistan

*Address all correspondence to: f.kushanov@genomics.uz; fakhriddinkushanov@gmail.com

References

[1] Higgins R, Thurber C, Assaranurak I, Brown P. Multiparental mapping of plant height and flowering time QTL in partially isogenic sorghum families. G3: Genes, Genomes. Genetics. 2014;**4**:1593-1602

[2] Horsfall JG. The fire brigade stops a raging corn epidemic. In: Hayes J, editor. The 1975 Yearbook of a Agriculture: That We May Eat. Washington DC: US Gov; 1975. pp. 105-114

[3] Fukunaga K, Hill J, Vigouroux Y, Matsuoka Y, Sanchez GJ, Liu K, et al. Genetic diversity and population structure of teosinte. Genetics. 2005;**169**(4):2241-2254

[4] Bennetzen JL. Maize genome structure and evolution. In: Bennetzen JL, Hake S, editors. Handbook of Maize: Genetics and Genomics. Berlin, Germany: Springer; 2009. pp. 179-199

[5] Liu Y, Wang L, Sun C, Zhang Z, Zheng Y, Qiu F. Genetic analysis and major QTL detection for maize kernel size and weight in multi-environments. Theoretical and Applied Genetics. 2014;**127**(5):1019-1037

[6] Randolph LF. Some effects of high temperature on polyploidy and other variations in maize. Proceedings of the National Academy of Science USA. 1932;**18**:222-229

[7] Shahzad AN, Pitann B, Ali H, Qayyum MF, Fatima A, Bakhat HF. Maize genotypes differing in salt resistance vary in jasmonic acid accumulation during the first phase of salt stress. Journal of Agronomy and Crop Science. 2015;**201**:443-451

[8] Liu J, Fernie AR, Yan J. The past, present, and future of maize improvement: Domestication, genomics, and functional genomic routes toward crop enhancement. Plant Communication. 2019;**1**(1):100010

[9] McClintock B. The production of homozygous deficient tissues with mutant characteristics by means of the aberrant mitotic behavior of ring-shaped chromosomes. Genetics. 1938;**23**(4):315-376

[10] Gaut BS, Doebley JF. DNA sequence evidence for the segmental allotetraploid origin of maize. Proceedings of the National Academy of Sciences. 1997;**94**(13):6809-6814. DOI: 10.1073/pnas.94.13.6809

[11] Liller CB, Walla A, Boer MP, et al. Fine mapping of a major QTL for awn length in barley using a multiparent mapping population. Theoretical and Applied Genetics. 2017;**130**:269-281

[12] Brandolini A. Razze europee di mais. Maydica. 1970;**15**:5-27

[13] Harpstead DD. Man-molded cereal: Hybrid corn's story. In: Hayes J, editor. The 1975 Yearbook of Agriculture: That We May Eat. Washington DC: US Gov; 1975. pp. 213-224

[14] Ranere, A. J.; Piperno, D. R.; Holst, I.; Dickau, R.; Iriarte, J. (2009). The cultural and chronological context of early Holocene maize and squash domestication in the Central Balsas River Valley, Mexico. Proceedings of the National Academy of Sciences 106(13):5014-5018; Anthony Ranere, Dolores Piperno et al. The cultural and chronological context of early Holocene maize and squash domestication in the Central Balsas River Valley, Mexcio. PNAS, March 24, 2009

[15] Callaway E. Shrub genome reveals secrets of flower power. Nature. 2013

[16] Gangurde SS, Kumar R, Pandey AK, Burow M, Laza HE, Nayak SN, et al.

Climate-smart groundnuts for achieving high productivity and improved quality: current status, challenges, and opportunities. In: Kole C, editor. Genomic Designing of Climate-Smart Oilseed Crops. Cham: Springer Nature Switzerland AG; 2019. pp. 133-172

[17] Li L, Briskine R, Schaefer R, Schnable P, Myers C, Flagel L, et al. Co-expression network analysis of duplicate genes in maize (*Zea mays* L.) reveals no subgenome bias. BMC Genomics. 2016;**17**:875

[18] Heslop-Harrison JS. Polyploidy. In: Maloy S, Hughes K, editors. Brenner's Encyclopedia of Genetics (Second Edition). San Diego, US: Academic Press; 2013. pp. 402-403. DOI: 10.1016/B978-0-12-374984-0.01192-X

[19] Niazi IAK, Rauf S, Teixeira da Silva JA, Iqbal Z, Munir H. Induced polyploidy in inter-subspecific maize hybrids to reduce heterosis breakdown and restore reproductive fertility. Grass and Forage Science. 2015;**70**(4):682-694

[20] Iqbal MZ, Cheng M, Zhao Y, Wen X, Zhang P, Zhang L, et al. Mysterious meiotic behavior of autopolyploid and allopolyploid maize. Comparative Cytogenetics. 2018;**12**(2):247-265

[21] Kushanov FN, Turaev OS, Ernazarova DK, Gapparov BM, Oripova BB, Kudratova MK, et al. Genetic diversity, QTL mapping, and marker-assisted selection technology in cotton (*Gossypium* spp.). Frontiers in Plant Science. 2021;**12**:779386

[22] Wu X, Chen F, Zhao X, Pang C, Shi R, Liu C, et al. QTL mapping and GWAS reveal the genetic mechanism controlling soluble solids content in *Brassica napus* shoots. Food. 2021;**10**:2400

[23] Guo J, Li C, Zhang X, Li Y, Zhang D, Shi Y, et al. Transcriptome and GWAS analyses reveal candidate gene for seminal root length of maize seedlings under drought stress. Plant Science. 2020;**292**:110380

[24] Edwards D, Batley J, Snowdon RJ. Accessing complex crop genomes with next-generation sequencing. Theoretical and Applied Genetics. 2013;**126**:1-11. DOI: 10.1007/s00122-012-1964-x

[25] Xiao Y, Liu H, Wu L, Warburton M, Yan J. Genome-wide association studies in maize: Praise and stargaze. Molecular Plant. 2017;**10**(3):359-374

[26] Luo M, Zhang Y, Li J, et al. Molecular dissection of maize seedling salt tolerance using a genome-wide association analysis method. Plant Biotechnology Journal. 2021;**19**(10):1937-1951. DOI: 10.1111/pbi.13607

[27] Xie Y, Feng Y, Chen Q, Zhao F, Zhou S, Ding Y, et al. Genome-wide association analysis of salt tolerance QTLs with SNP markers in maize (*Zea mays* L.). Genes Genomics. 2019;**41**(10):1135-1145

[28] Yuan J, Wang X, Zhao Y, et al. Genetic basis and identification of candidate genes for salt tolerance in rice by GWAS. Scientific Reports. 2020;**10**:9958

[29] Liu M, Tan X, Yang Y, Liu P, Zhang X, Zhang Y, et al. Analysis of the genetic architecture of maize kernel size traits by combined linkage and association mapping. Plant Biotechnology Journal. 2020;**18**:207-221

[30] Wang X, Wang H, Liu S, et al. Genetic variation in ZmVPP1 contributes to drought tolerance in maize seedlings. Nature Genetics. 2016;**48**:1233-1241

[31] Yuan Y, Cairns JE, Babu R, Gowda M, Makumbi D, Magorokosho C, et al. Genome-wide association mapping and genomic prediction

analyses reveal the genetic architecture of grain yield and flowering time under drought and heat stress conditions in maize. Frontiers in Plant Science. 2019;**9**:1919

[32] Dai LQ, Wu L, Dong QS, Yan G, Qu J, Wang PW. Genome-wide association analysis of maize kernel length. Journal of Northwest A&F University (Natural Science). 2018;**46**:20-28

[33] Liu S, Wang X, Wang H, Xin H, Yang X, Yan J, et al. Genome-wide analysis of ZmDREB genes and their association with natural variation in drought tolerance at seedling stage of Zea mays L. PLoS Genetics. 2013;**9**: e1003790

[34] Liu L, Du Y, Shen X, Li M, Sun W, Huang J, et al. KRN4 controls quantitative variation in maize kernel row number. PLoS Genetics. 2015;**11**: e1005670

[35] Zhang S, Thakare D, Yadegari R. Laser-capture microdissection of maize kernel compartments for RNA-Seq-based expression analysis. Methods in Molecular Biology. 2018;**1676**:153-163

[36] Zheng Y, Yuan F, Huang Y, et al. Genome-wide association studies of grain quality traits in maize. Scientific Reports. 2021;**11**:9797

[37] Liu Y, Yi Q, Hou X, et al. Identification of quantitative trait loci for kernel-related traits and the heterosis for these traits in maize (*Zea mays* L.). Molecular Genetics and Genomics. 2020;**295**:121-133

[38] Wang G, Zhao Y, Mao W, Ma X, Su C. QTL analysis and fine mapping of a major QTL conferring kernel size in maize (*Zea mays*). Frontiers in Genetics. 2020;**11**:603920

[39] Pan L, Wang N, Wu Z, Guo R, Yu X, Zheng Y, et al. A high density genetic map derived from RAD sequencing and its application in QTL analysis of yield-related traits in *Vigna unguiculata*. Frontiers in Plant Science. 2017;**8**:1544

[40] Li M, Guo X, Zhang M, Wang X, Zhang G, Tian Y, et al. Mapping QTLs for grain yield and yield components under high and low phosphorus treatments in maize (*Zea mays* L.). 2010;**178**(5):462

[41] Jiang GL. Molecular markers and marker-assisted breeding in plants. In: Andersen SB, editor. Plant Breeding from Laboratories to Fields. Rijeka, Croatia: IntechOpen; 2013. pp. 45-83

[42] Jiang Q, Tang D, Hu C, Qu J, Liu J. Combining meta-QTL with RNA-seq data to identify candidate genes of kernel row number trait in maize. Maydica. 2016;**61**:1-9

[43] Yu J, Holland JB, McMullen MD, Buckler ES. Genetic design and statistical power of nested association mapping in maize. Genetics. 2008;**78**(1):539-551

[44] Buckler ES, Holland JB, Bradbury PJ, Acharya CB, Brown PJ, Browne C, et al. The genetic architecture of maize flowering time. Science. 2009;**325**(5941):714-718

[45] McMullen MD, Kresovich S, Villeda HS, Bradbury P, Li H, Sun Q, et al. Genetic properties of the maize nested association mapping population. Science. 2009;**325**(737):737-740

[46] Bauer E et al. Intraspecific variation of recombination rate in maize. Genome Biology. 2013;**14**:R103

[47] Li H, Bowling AJ, Gandra P, et al. Systemic RNAi in western corn rootworm, Diabrotica virgifera virgifera, does not involve transitive pathways. Insect Science. 2018;**25**(1): 45-56. DOI: 10.1111/1744-7917.12382

[48] Chen Q et al. TeoNAM: A nested association mapping population for domestication and agronomic trait analysis in maize. Genetics. 2019;**213**:1065-1078

[49] Bouchet S, Olatoye MO, Marla SR, Perumal R, Tesso T, Yu J, et al. Increased power to dissect adaptive traits in global sorghum diversity using a nested association mapping population. Genetics. 2017;**206**:573-585

[50] Jordan DR, Mace ES, Cruickshank AW, Hunt CH, Henzell RG. Exploring and exploiting genetic variation from unadapted sorghum germplasm in a breeding program. Crop Science. 2011;**51**:1444-1457

[51] Mace ES, Hunt CH, Jordan DR. Supermodels: Sorghum and maize provide mutual insight into the genetics of flowering time. Theoretical and Applied Genetics. 2013 May;**126**(5):1377-1395

[52] Gangurde SS, Wang H, Yaduru S, Pandey MK, Fountain JC, Chu Y, et al. Nested-association mapping (NAM)-based genetic dissection uncovers candidate genes for seed and pod weights in peanut (Arachis hypogaea). Plant Biotechnology Journal. 2020 Jun;**18**(6):1457-1471. DOI: 10.1111/pbi.13311. [Epub Dec 25, 2019]. PMID: 31808273; PMCID: PMC7206994

[53] Gaut BS, Le Thierry d'Ennequin M, Peek AS, Sawkins MC. Maize as a model for the evolution of plant nuclear genomes. Proceedings of the National Academy of Sciences. 2000;**97**(13): 7008-7015. DOI: 10.1073/pnas. 97.13.7008

[54] Hemshrot A, Poets AM, Tyagi P, Lei L, Carter CK, Hirsch CN, et al. Development of a multiparent population for genetic mapping and allele discovery in six-row barley. Genetics. 2019;**213**:595-613

[55] Maurer A, Draba V, Jiang Y, et al. Modelling the genetic architecture of flowering time control in barley through nested association mapping. BMC Genomics. 2015;**16**:290

[56] Nice LM, Steffenson BJ, Brown-Guedira GL, Akhunov ED, Liu C, Kono TJY, et al. Development and genetic characterization of an advanced backcross-nested association mapping (AB-NAM) population of wild × cultivated barley. Genetics. 2016;**203**:1453-1467

[57] Schnaithmann F, Kopahnke D, Pillen K. A first step toward the development of a barley NAM population and its utilization to detect QTLs conferring leaf rust seedling resistance. Theoretical and Applied Genetics. 2014;**127**:1513-1525

[58] Schmutzer T, Samans B, Dyrszka E, et al. Species-wide genome sequence and nucleotide polymorphisms from the model allopolyploid plant *Brassica napus*. Sci Data. 2015;**2**:150072

[59] Bajgain P, Rouse MN, Tsilo TJ, Macharia GK, Bhavani S, Jin Y, et al. Nested association mapping of stem rust resistance in wheat using genotyping by sequencing. PLoS One. 2016;**11**:1-22

[60] Chidzanga C, Fleury D, Baumann U, Mullan D, Watanabe S, Kalambettu P, et al. Development of an Australian Bread Wheat Nested Association Mapping Population, a new genetic diversity resource for breeding under dry and hot climates. International Journal of Molecular Sciences. 2021;**22**:4348

[61] Jordan KW, Wang S, He F, Chao S, Lun Y, Paux E, et al. The genetic architecture of genome-wide recombination rate variation in allopolyploid wheat revealed by nested association mapping. The Plant Journal. 2018 Sep;**95**(6):1039-1054

[62] Kidane YG, Gesesse CA, Hailemariam BN, Desta EA,

Mengistu DK, Fadda C, et al. A large nested association mapping population for breeding and quantitative trait locus mapping in Ethiopian durum wheat. Plant Biotechnology Journal. 2019;**17**:1380-1393

[63] Wingen LU, West C, Leverington-Waite M, Collier S, Orford S, Goram R, et al. Wheat landrace genome diversity. Genetics. 2017;**205**(4):1657-1676. DOI: 10.1534/genetics.116.194688

[64] Christopher AF, Moreno M, Wang Z, Heffelfinger C, Arbelaez LJ, Aguirre JA, et al. Genetic architecture of a rice nested association mapping population. G3 Genes|Genomes|Genetics. 2017;**7**(6):1913-1926

[65] Kitony JK, Sunohara H, Tasaki M, Mori J-I, Shimazu A, Reyes VP, et al. Development of an Aus-derived nested association mapping (Aus-NAM) population in rice. Plants. 2021;**10**:1255

[66] Song J, Lu D, Niu Y, Sun H, Zhang P, Dong W, et al. Label-free quantitative proteomics of maize roots from different root zones provides insight into proteins associated with enhance water uptake. BMC Genomics. 2022;**23**(1):184

[67] Xavier A, Xu S, Muir WM, Rainey KM. NAM: Association studies in multiple populations. Bioinformatics. 2015;**31**:3862-3864

[68] Abdurakhmonov I, Abdullaev A, Buriev Z, Shermatov S, Kushanov F, Makamov A, et al. Cotton germplasm collection of Uzbekistan. In: Abdurakhmonov I, editor. World Cotton Germplasm Resources. London: IntechOpen; 2014

[69] Turaev O, Kushanov F, Makamov A, Darmonov M, Husenov N, Rakhmanov B. Statistical analysis for stability of fiber quality traits of cotton NAM founders. In: Proceedings of the III Tashkent International Innovation Forum. 2017. pp. 176-182

[70] Li H, Bradbury P, Ersoz E, Buckler ES, Wang J. Joint QTL linkage mapping for multiple-cross mating design sharing one common parent. PLoS One. 2011;**6**:e0017573

[71] Brock MT, Rubin MJ, DellaPenna D, Weinig C. A nested association mapping panel in *Arabidopsis thaliana* for mapping and characterizing genetic architecture. G3 Genes|Genomes|Genetics. 2020;**10**(10):3701-3708

[72] Scott MF, Ladejobi O, Amer S, et al. Multi-parent populations in crops: A toolbox integrating genomics and genetic mapping with breeding. Heredity. 2020;**125**:396-416

[73] Bevan H, Klara V, Arunas V, Chitra R, Vikas S, Pooran G, et al. MAGIC populations in crops: Current status and future prospects. Theoretical and Applied Genetics. 2015;**128**(6):999-1017. DOI: 10.1007/s00122-015-2506-0

[74] Mott R, Talbot CJ, Turri MG, Collins AC, Flint J. A method for fine mapping quantitative trait loci in outbred animal stocks. Proceedings of the National Academy of Sciences. 2000;**97**(23):12649-12654

[75] Cavanagh C, Morell M, Mackay I, Powell W. From mutations to MAGIC: Resources for gene discovery, validation and delivery in crop plants. Current Opinion in Plant Biology. 2008;**11**:215-221

[76] Mackay IJ, Powell W. The significance and relevance of linkage disequilibrium and association mapping in crops. Trends in Plant Science. 2007;**12**:53

[77] Kover PX, Valdar W, Trakalo J, Scarcelli N, Ehrenreich IM, et al. A multiparent advanced generation inter-cross to fine-map quantitative traits in *Arabidopsis thaliana*. PLoS Genetics. 2009;**5**(7):e1000551

[78] Anderson SL, Mahan AL, Murray SC, Klein PE. Four Parent Maize (FPM) population: Effects of mating designs on linkage disequilibrium and mapping quantitative traits. The Plant Genome. 2018;**11**(2). DOI: 10.3835/plantgenome2017.11.0102

[79] Dell'Acqua M, Gatti DM, Pea G, et al. Genetic properties of the MAGIC maize population: A new platform for high definition QTL mapping in *Zea mays*. Genome Biology. 2015;**16**:167

[80] Mahan AL, Murray SC, Klein PE. Four-parent maize (FPM) population: Development and phenotypic characterization. Crop Science. 2018;**58**:1106-1117

[81] Abdurakhmonov IY, Ayubov MS, Ubaydullaeva KA, Buriev ZT, Shermatov SE, Ruziboev HS, et al. RNA interference for functional genomics and improvement of cotton (*Gossypium* sp.). Frontiers in Plant Science. 2016;**22**(7):202

[82] Dalakouras A, Wassenegger M, Dadami E, Ganopoulos I, Pappas ML, Papadopoulou K. Genetically modified organism-free RNA interference: Exogenous application of RNA molecules in plants. Plant Physiology. 2020;**182**(1):38-50

[83] Segal G, Song R, Messing J. A new opaque variant of maize by a single dominant RNA-interference-inducing transgene. Genetics. 2003;**165**:387-397

[84] Casati P, Stapleton AE, Blum JE, Walbot V. Genome-wide analysis of high-altitude maize and gene knockdown stocks implicates chromatin remodeling proteins in response to UV-B. The Plant Journal. 2006 May;**46**(4):613-627

[85] Casati P, Walbot V. Maize lines expressing RNAi to chromatin remodeling factors are similarly hypersensitive to UV-B radiation but exhibit distinct transcriptome responses. Epigenetics. 2008;**3**(4):216-229

[86] Thakare D, Zhang J, Wing RA, Cotty PJ, Schmidt MA. Aflatoxin-free transgenic maize using host-induced gene silencing. Science Advances. 2017;**3**(3):e1602382

[87] Vélez AM, Fishilevich E, Rangasamy M, Khajuria C, McCaskill DG, Pereira AE, et al. Control of western corn rootworm via RNAi traits in maize: Lethal and sublethal effects of Sec23 dsRNA. Pest Management Science. Apr 2020;**76**(4):1500-1512. DOI: 10.1002/ps.5666

[88] Metje-Sprink J, Menz J, Modrzejewski D, Sprink T. DNA-free genome editing: Past, present and future. Frontiers in Plant Science. 2019;**9**:1957

[89] Nayak SN, Aravind B, Malavalli SS, Sukanth BS, Poornima R, Bharati P, et al. Omics technologies to enhance plant based functional foods: An overview. Frontiers in Genetics. 2021;**8**(12):742095

[90] D'Halluin K, Ruiter R. Directed genome engineering for genome optimization. The International Journal of Developmental Biology. 2013;**57**:621-627

[91] Shukla V, Doyon Y, Miller J, et al. Precise genome modification in the crop species *Zea mays* using zinc-finger nucleases. Nature. 2009;**459**:437-441

[92] Liang Z, Zhang K, Chen KL, Gao CX. Targeted mutagenesis in *Zea mays* using TALENs and the CRISPR/Cas system. Journal of Genetics and Genomics. 2014;**41**(2):63-68

[93] Char SN, Unger-Wallace E, Frame B, Briggs SA, Main M, Spalding MH, et al. Heritable site-specific mutagenesis using TALENs in maize. Plant Biotechnology Journal. 2015;**13**(7):1002-1010

[94] Malzahn A, Lowder L, Qi Y. Plant genome editing with TALEN and CRISPR. Cell & Bioscience. 2017;**7**:21

[95] Kubota C. Growth, Development, Transpiration and Translocation as Affected by Abiotic Environmental Factors. In: Kozai T, Niu G, Takagaki M, editors. Plant Factory: An Indoor Vertical Farming System for Efficient Quality Food Production. London, UK: Elsevier Inc.; 2015. pp. 151-164. DOI: 10.1016/B978-0-12-801775-3.00010-X

[96] Goff SA. A unifying theory for general multigenic heterosis: Energy efficiency, protein metabolism, and implications for molecular breeding. The New Phytologist. 2011;**189**(4):923-937

[97] Song Q et al. Genetic characterization of the soybean nested association mapping population. Plant Genome. 2017;**10**:1-14

[98] Pechanova O, Takáč T, Samaj J, Pechan T. Maize proteomics: An insight into the biology of an important cereal crop. Proteomics. 2013;**13**(3-4):637-662

[99] Eldakak M, Milad SI, Nawar AI, Rohila JS. Proteomics: A biotechnology tool for crop improvement. Frontiers in Plant Science. 2013;**4**:35

[100] Flores I, Cabra V, Quirasco MC, Farres A, Galvez A. Emulsifying properties of chemically deamidated corn (*Zea mays*) gluten meal. Food Science and Technology International. 2010;**16**(3):241-250

[101] Hochholdinger F, Marcon C, Baldauf JA, Yu P, Frey FP. Proteomics of maize root development. Frontiers in Plant Science. 2018;**9**:143

[102] Usuda H, Shimogawara K. Phosphate deficiency in maize. VI. Changes in the two-dimensional electrophoretic patterns of soluble proteins from second leaf blades associated with induced senescence. Plant & Cell Physiology. 1995;**36**:1149-1155

[103] Venkatesh TV, Chassy AW, Fiehn O, Flint-Garcia S, Zeng Q, Skogerson K, et al. Metabolomic assessment of key maize resources: GC-MS and NMR profiling of grain from B73 hybrids of the Nested Association Mapping (NAM) Founders and of geographically diverse landraces. Journal of Agricultural and Food Chemistry. 2016;**64**(10):2162-2172

[104] Zhang X, Zhang R, Li L, Yang Y, Ding Y, Guan H, et al. Negligible transcriptome and metabolome alterations in RNAi insecticidal maize against Monolepta hieroglyphica. Plant Cell Reports. 2020;**39**(11):1539-1547

[105] Khanna P, Kaur K, Gupta AK. Salicylic acid induces differential antioxidant response in spring maize under high temperature stress. Indian Journal of Experimental Biology. 2016;**54**(6):386-393

[106] Wu LJ, Zu XF, Wang XT, Sun AG, Zhang J, Wang SX, et al. Comparative proteomic analysis of the effects of salicylic acid and abscisic acid on maize (*Zea mays* L.) leaves. Plant Molecular Biology Reporter. 2013;**31**:507-516

[107] Mladenov V, Fotopoulos V, Kaiserli E, Karalija E, Maury S, Baranek M, et al. Deciphering the epigenetic alphabet involved in transgenerational stress memory in crops. International Journal of Molecular Sciences. 2021;**22**(13):7118

[108] Huang J, Lynn JS, Schulte L, Vendramin S, McGinnis K. Epigenetic control of gene expression in maize. International Review of Cell and Molecular Biology. 2017;**328**:25-48

[109] McClintock B. The origin and behavior of mutable loci in maize. Proceedings of the National Academy of Sciences of the United States of America. 1950;**36**(6):344-355

[110] Ding H, Gao J, Qin C, et al. The dynamics of DNA methylation in maize

roots under Pb stress. International Journal of Molecular Sciences. 2014;**15**(12):23537-23554

[111] Eichten SR, Swanson-Wagner RA, Schnable JC, et al. Heritable epigenetic variation among maize inbreds. PLoS Genetics. 2011;**7**(11):e1002372

[112] Forestan C, Farinati S, Aiese Cigliano R, et al. Maize RNA PolIV affects the expression of genes with nearby TE insertions and has a genome-wide repressive impact on transcription. BMC Plant Biology. 2017;**17**:161

[113] Gent JI, Madzima TF, Bader R, Kent MR, Zhang X, Stam M, et al. Accessible DNA and relative depletion of H3K9me2 at maize loci undergoing RNA-directed DNA methylation. The Plant Cell. 2014;**26**(12):4903-4917

[114] Li Q, Suzuki M, Wendt J, Patterson N, Eichten S, Hermanson P, et al. Post-conversion targeted capture of modified cytosines in mammalian and plant genomes. Nucleic Acids Research. 2015;**43**:e81

[115] Wang QX, Xie WB, Xing KJ, Yan J, Meng XJ, Li XL, et al. Genetic architecture of natural variation in rice chlorophyll content revealed by a genome-wide association study. Molecular Plant. 2015;**8**:946-957

[116] Regulski M, Lu Z, Kendall J, et al. The maize methylome influences mRNA splice sites and reveals widespread paramutation-like switches guided by small RNA. Genome Research. 2013;**23**(10):1651-1662

[117] West PT, Li Q, Ji L, Eichten SR, Song J, Vaughn MW, et al. Genomic distribution of H3K9me2 and DNA methylation in a maize genome. PLoS One. 2014;**9**(8):e105267

[118] Kravets O, Sokolova DO. Epigenetic factors of individual radiosensitivity and adaptive capacity. International Journal of Radiation Biology. 2020;**96**:1-29

[119] Han T, Wang F, Song Q, Ye W, Liu T, Wang L, et al. An epigenetic basis of inbreeding depression in maize. Science Advances. 2021;7(35):eabg5442

Chapter 5

Cotton as a Model for Polyploidy and Fiber Development Study

Venera S. Kamburova, Ilkhom B. Salakhutdinov, Shukhrat E. Shermatov, Zabardast T. Buriev and Ibrokhim Y. Abdurakhmonov

Abstract

Cotton is one of the most important crops in the world. The *Gossypium* genus is represented by 50 species, divided into two levels of ploidy: diploid (2n = 26) and tetraploid (2n = 52). This diversity of *Gossypium* species provides an ideal model for studying the evolution and domestication of polyploids. In this regard, studies of the origin and evolution of polyploid cotton species are crucial for understanding the ways and mechanisms of gene and genome evolution. In addition, studies of polyploidization of the cotton genome will allow to more accurately determine the localization of QTLs that determine fiber quality. In addition, due to the fact that cotton fibers are single trichomes originating from epidermal cells, they are one of the most favorable model systems for studying the molecular mechanisms of regulation of cell and cell wall elongation, as well as cellulose biosynthesis.

Keywords: cotton, polyploidy, genome evolution, cotton fiber, cell elongation

1. Introduction

Currently, the cotton (*Gossypium* L.) is one of the most important textile crops in the world, producing natural and quality fiber. For example, in 2017/18, the cotton world production and use were estimated at 25.1 million tons [1, 2]. As predicted, world cotton production will grow and reaching 26.1 million tons in 2026 [3].

The *Gossypium* genus is represented by more than 50 species, divided after ploidy into two groups: diploid (2n = 2x = 26) and tetraploid (2n = 4x = 52) [1, 4]. Moreover, 45 of species are diploid, and five remained species are tetraploid [4]. Among them, the diploid species such as *G. arboretum* L., *G. herbaceum* L. and tetraploid *G. hirsutum* L. and *G. barbadense* L. are cultivated only [4, 5]. Consequently, this kind of diversity of *Gossypium* species is a suitable model for studying the evolution, domestication and polyploidy, also to study of ploidy effect on the most important agronomic traits of cotton (e.g. fiber quality), as well as the expression and inheritance of corresponding genes of interest [6].

Similar to most plants, the evolution of cotton was characterized by repeating cycles of whole genome duplication [1, 6, 7]. At the same time, a parallel level of cytogenetic and genomic diversity emerged during the global widespread of the cotton, that finally led to the appearance of eight groups of diploid (n = 13) species (groups A-G and K of genomes) [1, 6]. It should be noted that despite the existence of different types of polyploidy [1, 6], the most common type is allopolyploidy, when two differentiated genomes, usually of various species, are combined in one cell nucleus as a result of hybridization [1, 6].

Thus, allopolyploid duplication of the genome leads to numerous of molecular genetic interactions, interlocus concerted evolution, difference of genomic evolution rates, interlocus transfer of genetic material, and possibly to changes in gene expression [1, 6]. In addition, allopolyploidy may have stimulated the morphological, ecological and physiological adaptation of cotton through natural selection based on a higher level of variability such as a result of duplication of the gene set [1, 6].

For the same reasons, the genome duplication may have given new opportunity for cotton improvement by directional selection [7, 8]. Another important aspect of allopolyploidy is that not every allopolyploid has to strictly correspond to concept of the simple summation of the ancestral diploid genomes. In some cases, the fusion of two different genomes is accompanied by significant genomic reorganization and non-Mendelian genetic inheritance as result [7, 9].

Consider to the mentioned above, we would attempt to analyze the consequences of evolution of polyploids, including on genomic, epigenomic and phenotypic levels in this chapter.

2. Evolution of *Gossypium* genus

According to molecular genetic data, the history of cotton evolution has amounted about 10–15 million years, after the *Gossypium* diverged from other *Gossypieae* [6, 10, 11]. In the same time, the evolution of eight groups of diploid species (genomic groups A-G and K) also occurred by the cotton widespread, that led to the arising of parallel level of cytogenetic and genomic diversity [1, 6, 11]. It should be noted that molecular genetic and cytogenetic studies show that the species lineages on genealogical tree of the genus coincide with genomic groups A-G, K, and AD and geographic origin [11, 12].

The evolution studies of the *Gossypium* have shown that the origination of tetraploid species proceeded by polyploidization of A- (African) and D-genomes (American) diploid species [1, 6, 11]. Alloploidization of these two genomes occurred about 1.5–2 million years ago, resulting in five different genomes: *G. darwinii*, *G. tomentosum*, *G. mustelinum*, *G. hirsutum* and *G. barbadense*, where the last two belong to cultivated species [13]. It was also proved that during the alloploidization process the *G. arboreum* and *G. herbaceum* were as receptors of A-genome and should be a predecessors, because all existing polyploid species contain the cytoplasm of the A genome. At the same time, the D-genome donor was appear *G. raimondii* [11].

After occurrence of the predecessor of allotetraploid species, at the initial stage of divergence led to the origination of two evolutionary lines of cotton with AD genomes: the first includes *G. mustelinum* (AD4 genome), the second one – all other species (AD1 – AD3 and AD5 genomes). In other words, the follow-up divergence of the second evolutionary line of AD genomes led to the emergence of recent allotetraploid cotton species such as *G. hirsutum* (AD1 genome), *G. barbadense* (AD2 genome), *G. tomentosum* (AD3 genome), and *G. darwinii* (AD5 genome) [11, 12].

One of an important evolutionary events for *Gossypium* was appear the domestication of four wild species. This selection was based on the length and quality of cotton fiber, which is anatomically specialized unicellular trichomes located on the surface of the epidermis of seeds [10, 11]. This sequential process led to the domestication of four species of cotton: two American – *G. hirsutum* and *G. barbadense* and two Afro-Asian – *G. arboretum* and *G. herbaceum* [11].

Followed phylogenetic studies have shown the trait of prolonged elongation of trichomes has appeared first time in the A/F-genomes. Possibly, it was the reason to domestication of *G. arboretum* and *G. herbaceum* (A-genome). Unlike A-genome a number of species with D-genome (*G. thurberi*, *G. trilobum*, *G. davidsonii* and *G. klotzschianum*, and three species of the *Cauducibracteolata* subsection) lack of clearly visible fibers [11, 12]. This suggests that the traits of prolongation of trichomes were probably inherited by the allotetraploid (AD-genome) from the A-genome [11].

Moreover, the domestication of cotton species led to a change not only in the length of the fiber, but also in the chemical composition of its: the fiber of wild species besides cellulose contains suberin, while in cultivated species it is cellulose only [11].

Summarizing the information mentioned above, it should be noted that the *Gossypium* diverged from other *Gossypieae* in the Pleistocene period eventualy. This genus has evolved in two ways: divergence at diploid species(genomic groups A-G and K) and allopolyploidization of A- and D-genomes, followed by arising of tetraploid species (AD1 - AD5-genomes). Besides this, the domestication of these species and artificial selection based on fiber quality have also greate influenced on evolution of cultivated cotton.

3. Mechanisms of polyploidy

Polyploidization of eukaryotic genomes is an important evolutionary event that had a significant effect on the evolution of plants, including cotton [14–16]. Polyploids are divided into two large groups: autopolyploids and allopolyploids [17–20]. The difference between these two groups basically lies in the hybridization type: intraspecific hybridization occurs in autopolyploids, while allopolyploids arise by the combination of processes such as interspecies hybridization and duplication of chromosomes [17, 20].

In turn, there are two types of allopolyploids: true and segmental allopolyploids. True allopolyploids emerged due to hybridization of distantly related species, but segmental allopolyploids through hybridization of closely related species with partially different genomes [20]. In this case, segmental allopolyploids can be considered as an intermediate type between true allopolyploids and autopolyploids [20].

In autopolyploids, the presence of more than two homologous chromosomes in the genome may lead to formation of multivalents during meiosis. It contributes to the polysomic type of inheritance of traits. Whereas, in true allopolyploids bivalents are formed, that leads to disomic inheritance of traits. At the same process, in segmental allopolyploids monovalent, bivalent and/or multivalent chromosome pairing is observed during meiosis [20].

The second mechanism is the fusion of unreduced gametes – the basic factor of the natural emergence of polyploidy. In this case, the fusion of unreduced gametes may lead to unilateral- (fusion with a typically reduced gamete) or bilateral polypolydization (fusion with another unreduced gamete) [20].

The formation of unreduced gametes can occur due to errors during meiosis. In this case, errors during meiosis I (first division restitution – FDR) can be a consequence of a fail to chromosome pairing in prophase I (synaptene/pachytene) or separation of homologous chromosomes in anaphase I [20]. At the same time, errors during meiosis II (second division restitution - SDR) occur in anaphase II due to the fail to separation and segregation of sister chromatids [20]. Both of FDR and SDR lead to a chromosome set doubling in gametes, resulted in dyads or triads formation [21].

Depending on the meiotic restitution mechanism, a polyploidization consequences will differ. Thus, after FDR, the heterozygosity level of unreduced gametes will be similar to the original gametes, while SDR leads to a decrease in the level of heterozygosity of unreduced gametes [20]. The heterozygosity level of a resulting polyploids will be of decisive importance both in the struggle for survival as well as by artificial selection.

Polyploidy had a significant effect on the evolution process and formation of species by increasing phenotypic variability, heterosis, and mutation resistance. On the other hand, in terms of evolution, allopolyploidization (interspecific hybridization) is more preferable due to the pronounced effect of heterosis, that manifest in increasing of biomass, growth and its rate, fertility and resistance of occured hybrids to stress [22]. Thus, in tetraploid cultivated cotton species (*G. hirsutum* and *G. barbadense*) the quality and yield of fiber are much higher than cultivated diploids (*G. arboretum* and *G. herbaceum*) [23].

Resuming the above, polyploidization is rather widespread phenomenon in plant evolution (the number of polyploid species is approximately ¼ of the total number of vascular plant species) [24]. At the same time, the polyploidy occurrence brings an evolutionary "benefit" to a species, increasing its chances in the struggle for survival.

4. Genomic consequences of polyploidization

The allopolyploidization process of cotton genome could not be considered as the simple sum of the A- and D-genomes. It has been shown that genome duplication leads to various molecular genetic interactions e.g.: interlocus consistent evolution, different rates of genomes evolution, interlocus transfer of genetic material and changes in gene expression [1, 6, 17].

Additionally, according to the latest molecular data tetraploid cotton species are at least paleo-octaploids, and diploid species are paleo-tetraploids. Due to this fact cotton may be a good model system for studying consequences of genome polyploidization [6, 9, 25].

In connection with the above, let us review the changes that occurred after polyploidization of the cotton genome.

4.1 Genome stability

Despite the fact that diploid Gossypium species have the same chromosome basic number (n = 13), the DNA length in different species widely varies from ~900 Mb in D-genomes to ~2500 Mb in K-genomes [1, 6, 17]. Moreover, the analysis of bivalents formation in the metaphase of meiosis also suggest that diploid cotton species are actually paleopolyploid organisms [6]. A number of studies have also shown that the ancestor of *Gossypium* went off through cycles of polyploidization, followed by the loss of a part of homologous genes and diploidization [6, 26, 27].

In this respect it should be noted that allopolyploidization of cotton has not only characterized by rearrangements at the chromosome level [1, 6]. This assumption was confirmed by both classical cytogenetic and molecular genetic data [1, 6]. Thus, cytogenetic data show that chromosomes of A- and D-genome less form bivalents after crossing of allotetraploids compared to diploid species hybrids [1, 6]. For example, hybrids of allotetraploids form less than one bivalent per cell in the meiotic metaphase, while hybrids of present diploids of A- as well as D-genome form, on average, 5.8 and 7.8 bivalents [1, 6].

Additionally, the analysis of the order and syntheny of genes in the A- and D-genomes as well as allopolyploid genomes (A versus At and D versus Dt) showed a low level of structural chromosome rearrangements with a retention of collinear linkage groups [28]. Along with this, AFLP analysis of nine artificial allotetraploid and allohexaploid cotton species showed a significant additivity of genetic loci [1, 6].

Summarizing the facts, it can be assumed that the cotton genome stabilization after polyploidization led to such reorganization of the original genomes that they were no longer able to homeological pairing [1, 6].

Thus, it can be concluding that the cotton genome is quite stable and genome stabilization is not achieved through structural rearrangements unlike some other plant models with polyploid genome.

4.2 Mobile elements in genome

As mentioned above, the genome size of different cotton species differs significantly even the same basic number of chromosomes [1, 6, 29]. This may be conditioned with a number mobile genetic elements (MGE) in the *Gossypium* genome [6]. Wu et al. (2017) have shown that the *Gossypium* genome contains a large number of MGE, particularly a long terminal repeat (LTR) retrotransposons in compare to *Theobroma cacao* (L.) and *A. thaliana* (L.) Heynh [30].

Moreover, the analysis of the genomes of *G. raimondii*, *G. arboreum*, and *G. hirsutum* showed that the greatest number of MGE, especially LTR-retrotransposons is observed in A- and AD-genome [6, 12, 31, 32]. However, the frequency of occurrence of *Copia* LTR retrotransposons is higher in *G. raimondii* (D5 genome) – the smallest genome size (885 Mb). At the same time, the occurrence frequency of the *Gypsy* LTR retroelements is higher in species with a large genome size [6, 32–34]. Additionally, it was established that the wide distribution of *GORGE3* (*Gossypium* retrotransposable *gypsy*-like element) in A- and AD-genome was the reason for their upsizing [31, 32, 35, 36].

It has been also found that besides the genome resizing in various cotton species, MGEs have also affected on the expression of genes responsible for fiber development [30, 32]. Thus, in D-subgenome was observed the insertion of the *Copia* LTR retrotransposon into promoter region of the gene encoding the transcription factor *GhMYB25*. This well consists with the facts of hyperexpression of the D-genome homeolog in *G. hirsutum* [32]. Similarly, the insertion of the LINE retrotransposon into promoter of ethylene response factor (*GhERF*) gene in D-subgenome increases the expression level of the D-homeologue in compare to its A-copy [32].

It has been also suggested that the silencing of CICR (Chinese Institute of Cotton Research) LTR elements had an appreciable effect on the formation of allotetraploid cotton species, because the occurrence frequency of these MGEs is significant in the A-subgenomes, and practically not occur in the D-subgenomes [37].

Summarize this, presence of mobile elements in a genome, their polymorphism and occurrence frequency, probably had the significant influence on the cotton evolution. In addition, MGE are involved in regulation of activity of genes responsible for fiber quality.

4.3 Asymmetric evolution of the genome

Hereof the *Gossypium* has both diploid and tetraploid genome, it makes cotton an ideal model to study of the homeologous genes evolution and their expression after polyploidization.

As mentioned above, the extended trichomes elongation trait was probably inherited by the allotetraploid AD-genomes from the A-genome [11]. Further evolution of domesticated tetraploids (*G. hirsutum* and *G. barbadense*) was done under the influence of artificial selection directed on improving fiber quality. Its led to the asymmetric evolution of the A- and D-subgenomes. According Li et al. (2015) in *G. hirsutum* the mutation frequency and formation rate of single nucleotide polymorphisms (SNPs) within intergenic collinear regions of the Dt-subgenome were significantly higher than in the At-genome [31]. Meanwhile, established Ks values for pairs of collinear genes in the At- and Dt-subgenomes were less than in the corresponding diploid A- and D-genomes. It was also shown reducing of dN/dS ratio in Dt/D pair in comparison with *T. cacao* and similar indicators for At/A [31].

In addition, scientists have found a greater extension of total rearrangements in At-subgenome (372.6 Mb) compared to Dt-subgenome (82.6 Mb) by comparative study of interchromosomal rearrangements and SNP frequency in *G. hirsutum* and *G. barbadense* [38]. It was also shown that SNP frequency is increased in the At-subgenome in both *G. hirsutum* and *G. barbadense* by comparing the Dt-subgenome (5.95 per thousand nucleotides in At-subgenome versus of 5.81 in the Dt-subgenome) [38].

These data also show that allotetraploid genomes due to genetic redundancy are being under less pressure from stabilizing selection, and directed selection by fiber quality has a greater effect on the At-subgenome [31, 38].

The asymmetry of these subgenomes is also appeared by the mutation types occurring in allotetraploid genomes of *G. hirsutum* and *G. barbadense*. Thus, it was found that duplications in the At-subgenome were more conserved than in the Dt-subgenome of *G. hirsutum*. At the same time, there are more conservative deletions in Dt-subgenome compared to the At-subgenome of *G. barbadense* [39]. These data indicate that artificial selection during cotton domestication furthered the fixation of duplications in the At-subgenome in *G. hirsutum*, and deletions in the Dt-subgenome of *G. barbadense*. It may have contributed to the development of a higher fiber quality in Pima cotton that distinguishes the species from others [39].

Differences in subgenomes are also manifested by different occurrence of frequency and activity of MGE. Two independent research groups have found that MGE number in At-subgenome exceeded the same parameter in Dt-subgenome [31, 40]. At the same time, the frequency of LTR-*Gypsy* occurrence in the At-subgenome was significantly higher than in the Dt-subgenome [31, 40]. Li et al. (2015) have also found that subgenomes differ not only in the MGEs number within them, but also by transcriptional activity and location [31]. Thus, it was shown that the transcription level of both LTR-*Copia* and LTR-*Gypsy* was increased in the Dt-subgenome compared with the At-subgenome [31]. However, LTR-*Copia* were more active and more frequently located near the coding genes when compared to LTR-*Gypsy* [16].

The asymmetry is also manifested in the unequal expression of At- or Dt-homeologs, which regulate fiber development in cotton [31, 41–43]. The expression level of homeologs of some transcription factors (eg, *MYB*) was significantly increased in the At-subgenome [31]. And the comprehensive proteomic analysis of the fiber of allopolyploid species (*G. hirsutum* and *G. barbadense*) have shown that A-patterns of expression prevailed in *G. hirsutum* over ones in *G. barbadense* at different stages of fiber development. Thus, the expression level changed the direction of dominance from D-genome to A-genome [42].

Moreover, the results obtained using the RNA-seq technology on *G. hirsutum* have shown a shift on the level of homeologs expression towards the A-subgenome in allotetraploid cotton [44]. This shift of gene expression can be explained by the deactivation of homeologs in non-dominant D-subgenome due to negative regulators (miRNA and transcriptional repressors) [6, 44]. It was also established that genes in A-subgenome may be responsible for the fiber development by regulation of fatty acids biosynthesis/metabolism and microtubules growing process. While the genes in D-subgenome may be involved to the transcription regulation and stress response [44].

Thus, the analysis of the available data allows to speak about the asymmetric evolution of allopolyploid cotton subgenomes with a shift in dominance towards A-subgenome.

5. Effects of polyploidy on fiber development

The fiber is one of the key point for domestication of four *Gossypium* species: two diploid *G. arboretum* and *G. herbaceum* (A-genome), as well as two tetraploid species *G. hirsutum* and *G. barbadense* (AD-genome) [11]. In the meantime, the domestication process of tetraploid species was independent, that have been confirmed both the sequencing data and significant differences in cotton fiber at the proteome level [42, 43, 45].

Cotton fiber is basically elongated single cell of seed epidermis (trichome) with a clear gradation of development stages: fiber initiation, elongation, secondary biosynthesis of the cell walls and maturation [33, 46, 47]. It first appeared among ancestral diploid cotton with A-genome after divergence with F-genome [1, 6, 48]. Allotetraploid species (AD genomes) have significantly higher fiber quality, that can be explained by the nucleotypic effect after allopolyploidization of A- and D-genome [48, 49].

Polyploidization has also led to increase of the number of nuclear genes associated with fiber development [47]. E.g., a number of studies have shown the content of Malvaceae specific genes of *MIXTA* family, encoding *MYB* transcription factors and regulating fiber development is significantly higher in allotetraploid species [50, 51]. Additionally, stabilization of the natural and artificial selection contributed a changes at the expression level of fiber development genes. It has been achieved either by epigenetic modifications (DNA methylation, miRNA and siRNA biogenesis) or by histones modification, among other factors [48, 52].

The fiber development in cotton is a complex process ensured by the coordinated action of many genes involvong to biosynthesis of polysaccharides, lipids and phytohormones, pro- and antioxidant system, calcium homeostasis, as well as transcription factor genes (*MYB, C2H2, bHLH, WRKY* and *HD-ZIP*) [40, 53–55]. At the same time, in tetraploid species, the expression and co-expression of genes at different stages of fiber development is different: some genes are expressed at the stage of fiber initiation, others - at the stages of fiber elongation and secondary cell walls biosynthesis [53, 54]. It has been shown that genes in the Dt-subgenome are predominantly expressed at the stage of fiber initiation, very important parameter to the fiber yield [1, 33].

The difference of gene expression level between *G. hirsutum* and *G. barbadense* was also established using whole genomes alighnment of both species. It was shown that a longer fiber of *G. barbadense* may be a result of more continuous activity of genes encoding sucrose transporter (*GbTSTl*), Na^+/H^+-antiporter (*GbNHXl*), aluminum-activated malate transporter (*GbALMT16*), vacuolar-localized vacuolar invertase (*GbVIN1*) and plasmodesmata (*PD*) [8].

It was also found that the fiber development in tetraploid is specified by gene expression in both At- and Dt-subgenome [1, 40, 48, 55]. Despite the fact that major genes for fiber quality were introduced into allopolyploids from A-genome, the genes in Dt-subgenome also take a significant effect on the fiber development in tetraploid cotton [48]. For example, several researchers on the base of an integrated genetic and physical map of fiber development genes supposed that a transcription factors regulating the expression of fiber genes in At-subgenome are transcribed in Dt-subgenome [1, 56].

Along with this, another research group has identified 811 positively selected genes (PSG) in *G. hirsutum*, 591 of them were associated with fiber development [40, 55]. Along with this, another research group has identified 811 positively selected genes (PSG) in *G. hirsutum*, 591 of them were associated with fiber development [40, 55]. Moreover, 58% of these PSGs were localized in At-subgenome, and 42% of PSGs were identified in the Dt-subgenome only. Moreover, it has been shown that PSGs in At-subgenome are associated with beta-D-glucan biosynthesis, regulation of signal transduction, as well as carbohydrates and sucrose biosynthesis. While, PSGs in Dt-subgenome determine the stress responses, which, as is known, reflect on fiber development [40, 55, 57].

All of these results were confirmed by studies of functional enrichment of proteins differentially expressed in cotton fiber [42]. The results of the study of proteome in *G. hirsutum* and *G. barbadense* have shown that the dominant expression pattern of *G. hirsutum* was more similar to A-genome (*G. arboretum*), while dominant expression pattern of *G. barbadense* was different dependent on fiber development stage, and switched from Dt- subgenome to At-subgenome [42]. In this case, the dominant patterns of At-subgenome produced the enzymes involved to biosynthesis of alcohols, monosaccharides and hexoses, while the patterns of Dt-subgenome produced proteins involved in various stress responses [42]. These results allowed to suggest that similarity in fiber appearance of these two species arose during evolution but through different pathways at the proteomic level [42].

The results obtained by genome sequencing of tetraploid *G. hirsutum* and diploid *G. arboretum* and *G. raimondii* have shown that difference of gene expression between *G. hirsutum* and *G. raimondii* was significantly higher than between *G. hirsutum* and *G. arboretum* [44]. It has been also demonstrated a shift of the expression level towards the At-subgenome, explained by the authors as an activation/deactivation of Dt-homeologs by negative regulators such as miRNA and transcription repressors. Deactivation of Dt homeologues was confirmed by a reduced number of nonfunctional genes in the Dt-subgenome [44]. The other authors have shown that the Dt-subgenome dominant pattern of *G. hirsutum* is associated with stress responses (genes encoding phosphatidylinositol phosphate kinase PIPK, PIP (internal plasma membrane protein), calmodulin (CaM), ethylene receptors and ethylene response factors (ERF), ABA receptors (PYR/PYL), protein kinase SnRK and protein kinase PP2C [8].

Thus, all of these data show that hybridization of A- and D-genome in allopolyploids had a significant effect on the fiber development in cotton due to both nucleotypic effect as well as changes and differentiation at the expression level of homeologuesof in At- and Dt-subgenome. Obviously, At-genes are associated with the fiber development, while Dt-genes regulate the activity of At-genes towards to fiber quality and determine the adaptive capabilities of allotetraploid cotton to adverse environment conditions [8, 42, 44].

6. Differential evolution of subgenomes

Following the fusion of two genomes into a single nucleus due to allopolyploidy, it is expected that some genes will acquire mutations and become pseudogenes, while others may diverge and acquire new functions [17–19]. However, it can be expected that these and other phenomena affecting the genes molecular evolution, will be equally distributed in the two allopoliploid genomes. This leads to a useful null hypothesis, that is, the evolutionary rates of nucleotide substitutions will be equivalent for duplicated homeologists [17–19]. This leads to the null hypothesis, according to which the evolutionary rates of nucleotide substitutions will be equivalent for duplicated homeologs [17–19]. Inference expectation is that both gene copies accumulate intraspecific diversity at equivalent rates. However, this is not always true, for example, when there is strong directional selection per gene copy [17–19]. However, in the presence of strong stabilizing selection per gene copy, this condition got broken [17–19].

Despite this, this model can be useful in study the mechanisms underlying differential evolutionary rates or different levels of diversity. Thus, if one of the homeolog becomes pseudogenized, while the others remain under the pressure of purifying selection, an increase in nucleotide diversity can be expected at a higher rate in the first locus than in the last one [15, 19]. Finding duplicated genes in the same nucleus simplifies the problem of isolating potentially important genomic forces from population-level factors that can influence diversity patterns, such as the selection system or effective population size [15, 19]. Since population factors are neutral in regards to the two homeologs, the observed differences in diversity are almost certainly associated with genetic or genomic processes [15, 17–19].

Gossypium allopolyploids is a suitable model for these studies, especially when the two genomes are largely collinear but genome size differ in twice [1, 14, 15, 58–60]. The assumption of unequal speeds evolution in A- and D-genomes was confirmed by the observations that synthetic A- and D-genomic hybrids may be formed only when the A genome is used as a recipient [6]. This phenomenon is confirmed by divergent indicators. Thus, the study of the levels of RFLP polymorphisms found in allopolyploid cotton has shown that the number of polymorphisms in the Dt-subgenome was greater than in the At-subgenome [1, 14, 15, 58–60]. Similarly, two independent phylogenetic analyzes allowed to find out that D-genomic sequences in allopolyploids have longer phylogenetic branches and higher evolutionary rates in comparison to their homeologous A-genomic sequences [1, 14, 58]. Moreover, localization of quantitative traits loci indicates higher rates of evolution in the D-subgenome [1, 14, 58–60].

In addition, a direct test of the null hypothesis of the nucleotide substitution rates equivalence for homeologous genes is provided by measuring of the levels of nucleotide diversity [1, 17–19]. If evolutionary forces are equal for duplicated genes, mutations must accumulate randomly towards the homeolog. Therefore, the number of detected alleles should be approximately equal for two gene copies in the study of allelic polymorphism [1, 17–19, 58]. This approach was used by researchers in the study of the nucleotide sequences of the alcohol dehydrogenase gene (*AdhA*) in *G. hirsutum* and *G. barbadense* [61]. In both allopolyploid species the estimates of nucleotide diversity were twice as high for the Dt-homeolog of *AdhA* gene [60]. Similar data were obtained in the study of other gene of alcohol dehydrogenase (*AdhC*) [62].

Thus, these data allowed to suggest the existence of the increasing rate of Dt-subgenome evolution of the allopolyploid *Gossypium*. In addition, the evolutionary forces affecting *Gossypium* subgenomes can be fundamentally different. At the same time, it should be noted that the molecular mechanisms underlying the differential evolution of subgenomes remain unclear. However, it is logical to assume that they are associated with a double difference in genomic size.

7. Conclusion and future prospect

Summarizing the aforementioned, due to *Gossypium* diversity including both diploid (2n = 2x = 26) and tetraploid (2n = 4x = 52) species, cotton may be an ideal model for studying the evolution of allopolyploids, as well as the influence of ploidy for the most important agronomic traits – cotton fiber quality [1, 6, 33, 55]. In addition, the presence four cultivated species (diploid - *G. arboretum* and *G. herbaceum* and tetraploid - *G. hirsutum* and *G. barbadense*) allow to use this plant as a model for studying the effect of artificial selection in domestication process to shift of the homeologous expression level in tetraploid towards one of the subgenome [1, 6, 33, 55]. Moreover, because of cotton fiber is a single and easily isolated cell with a clear gradated of developmental stages, it is a good model to study of fiber development mechanisms [47].

This chapter presents the results of research on the evolution of *Gossypium*, mechanisms of polyploidization, genomic consequences of polyploidy, including the role of mobile genetic elements and asymmetric expression of homeologues, as well as the polyploidy effect on fiber quality traits. These data clarify the evolution history of this genus and mechanisms that regulate the formation and elongation of fiber.

Despite the volume of the obtained data, there are many unsolved issues in cotton genomics. Thus, the study the subgenome asymmetry using LTR-elements will help to clarify the evolution of *Gossypium* genomes and their divergence in time. Analysis of MGE polymorphisms may help identify genes involving to development of cotton fiber.

In addition, the issues of sub- and neofunctionalization of duplicated genes remain unclear, as well as the mechanism and relationship of epigenetic regulation in asymmetric expression of homeologous genes.

Continuation of comparative transcriptome and proteomic studies will also make it possible to more accurately differentiate the of natural and artificial selection influence on cultivated cotton species. At the same time, these studies can be a good basis for a more complete characterization of the metabolic pathways underlying the fiber formation and development.

Such research as genotyping and more accurate assembly of reference genomes, pan-genomic approaches (sequencing of gene pool in a populations), big data analysis, genome editing, de-novo domestication and genomic selection, combined with the available data, will allow for more efficient development of new cotton varieties with the desired properties as well as developing of personalized farming technologies for this crop.

Author details

Venera S. Kamburova*, Ilkhom B. Salakhutdinov, Shukhrat E. Shermatov, Zabardast T. Buriev and Ibrokhim Y. Abdurakhmonov
Center of Genomics and Bioinformatics, Academy of Science of Republic of Uzbekistan, Tashkent, Uzbekistan

*Address all correspondence to: venera.k75@gmail.com

References

[1] Wendel JF, Flagel LE, Adams KL. Jeans, Genes, and Genomes: Cotton as a Model for Studying Polyploidy. In: Soltis P, Soltis D, editors. Polyploidy and Genome Evolution. Berlin: Springer; 2012. p. 181-207. DOI: 10.1007/978-3-642-31442-1_10

[2] Khan MA, Wahid A, Ahmad M, Tahir MT. World Cotton Production and Consumption: An Overview. In: Ahmad S, Hasanuzzaman M, editors. Cotton Production and Uses. Singapore: Springer Nature Singapore Pte Ltd; 2020. p. 1-7. DOI: 10.1007/978-981-15-1472-2_1

[3] Cotton [Internet]. Available from: http://www.fao.org/3/BT093e/BT093e.pdf

[4] Emani C. Transgenic Cotton for Agronomical Useful Traits. In: Ramawat K, Ahuja M, editors. Fiber Plants. Sustainable Development and Biodiversity. Vol. 13. Cham: Springer; 2016. p. 201-216. DOI: 10.1007/978-3-319-44570-0_10

[5] Sun Y, Zhang X, Huang C, Guo X, Nie Y. Somatic embryogenesis and plant regeneration from different wild diploid cotton (*Gossypium*) species. Plant Cell Rep. 2006;25:289-296. DOI: 10.1007/s00299-005-0085-2

[6] Strygina K, Khlestkina E, Podolnaya L. Cotton genome evolution and features of its structural and functional organization. Bio. Comm. 2020;65(1):15-27. DOI: 10.21638/spbu03.2020.102

[7] McGrath CL, Lynch M. Evolutionary Significance of Whole-Genome Duplication. In: Soltis P, Soltis D, editors. Polyploidy and Genome Evolution. Berlin: Springer; 2012. p. 1-20. DOI: 10.1007/978-3-642-31442-1_1

[8] Hu Y, Chen J, Fang L, et al. *Gossypium barbadense* and *Gossypium hirsutum* genomes provide insights into the origin and evolution of allotetraploid cotton. Nat Genet. 2019;51:739-748. DOI: 10.1038/s41588-019-0371-5

[9] Meng F, Pan Y, Wang J, Yu J, et al. Cotton Duplicated Genes Produced by Polyploidy Show Significantly Elevated and Unbalanced Evolutionary Rates, Overwhelmingly Perturbing Gene Tree Topology. Front. Genet. 2020;11:239. DOI: 10.3389/fgene.2020.00239

[10] Brubaker CL, Bourland FM, Wendel JF. The origin and domestication of cotton. In Smith CW, Cothren JT, editors. Cotton: Origin, History, Technology and Production. New York: Wiley; 1999. p. 3-31.

[11] Wendel JF, Brubaker C, Alvarez I, Cronn R, Stewart JM. Evolution and Natural History of the Cotton Genus. In: Paterson AH, editor. Genetics and Genomics of Cotton. Plant Genetics and Genomics: Crops and Models. Vol. 3. New York: Springer; 2009. p. 3-22. DOI: 10.1007/978-0-387-70810-2_1

[12] Kim, H. J. Fiber Biology. In: Fang DD, Percy RG, editors. Cotton, 2nd ed., Agron. Monogr. 57. Madison: ASA, CSSA, and SSSA; 2015. p. 97-128. DOI: 10.2134/agronmonogr57.2013.0022

[13] Abdurakhmonov IY, Buriev ZT, Shermatov SS, Abdullaev AA, Urmonov K, Kushanov F, et al. Genetic diversity in *Gossypium* genus. In Galiskan M, editor. Genetic diversity in Plants. Rijeka: InTech Press; 2012. p. 331-338. DOI: 10.5772/35384

[14] Wendel JF, Grover CE. Taxonomy and Evolution of the Cotton Genus, *Gossypium*. In: Fang DD, Percy RG, editors. Cotton, 2nd ed., Agron. Monogr. 57. Madison: ASA, CSSA,

and SSSA; 2015. p. 25-44. DOI: 10.2134/agronmonogr57.2013.0020

[15] Madlung A. Polyploidy and its effect on evolutionary success: old questions revisited with new tools. Heredity. 2013;110:99-104. DOI: 10.1038/hdy.2012.79

[16] Chen ZJ, Sreedasyam A, Ando A, et al. Genomic diversifications of five *Gossypium* allopolyploid species and their impact on cotton improvement. Nat Genet. 2020;52:525-533. DOI: 10.1038/s41588-020-0614-5

[17] Soltis PS. Hybridization in Plants. In Levin SA, editor. Encyclopedia of Biodiversity (Second Edition). Oxford: Academic Press; 2013. p. 166-176. DOI: 10.1016/b978-0-12-384719-5.00202-1

[18] Counterman BA. Hybrid Speciation. In Kliman RM, editor. Encyclopedia of Evolutionary Biology. Oxford: Academic Press; 2016. p. 242-248. DOI: 10.1016/b978-0-12-800049-6.00072-x

[19] Blackman BK. Speciation Genes. In Kliman RM, editor. Encyclopedia of Evolutionary Biology. Oxford: Academic Press; 2016. p. 166-175. DOI: 10.1016/b978-0-12-800049-6.00066-4

[20] Sattler MC, Carvalho CR, Clarindo WR. The polyploidy and its key role in plant breeding. Planta. 2016;243:281-296. DOI: 10.1007/s00425-015-2450-x

[21] Ramanna MS, Jacobsen E. Relevance of sexual polyploidization for crop improvement: a review. Euphytica. 2003;133:3-8. DOI: 10.1023/A:1025600824483

[22] Chen ZJ. Molecular mechanisms of polyploidy and hybrid vigor. Trends Plant Sci. 2010;15:57-72. DOI: 10.1016/j.tplants.2009.12.003

[23] Renny-Byfield S, Wendel JF. Doubling down on genomes: polyploidy and crop plants. Am J Bot. 2014;101: 1-15. DOI: 10.3732/ajb.1400119

[24] Barker MS, Arrigo N, Baniaga AE, Li Z, Levin DA. On the relative abundance of autopolyploids and allopolyploids. New Phytol. 2016;210(2):391-398. DOI: 10.1111/nph.13698

[25] Renny-Byfeld S, Gong L, Gallagher JP, Wendel JF. Persistence of subgenomes in paleopolyploid cotton after 60 my of evolution. Molecular Biology and Evolution. 2015;32(4):1063-1071. DOI: 10.1093/molbev/msv001

[26] Renny-Byfeld S, Gallagher JP, Grover CE, Szadkowski E, et al. Ancient gene duplicates in *Gossypium* (cotton) exhibit near-complete expression divergence. Genome Biology and Evolution. 2014;6(3):559-571. DOI: 10.1093/gbe/evu037

[27] Birchler J.A. Genetic Consequences of Polyploidy in Plants. In: Soltis P, Soltis D, editors. Polyploidy and Genome Evolution. Berlin: Springer; 2012. p. 21-32. DOI: 10.1007/978-3-642-31442-1_2

[28] Zhang T, Endrizzi JE. Cytology and Cytogenetics. In: Fang DD, Percy RG, editors. Cotton, 2nd ed., Agron. Monogr. 57. Madison: ASA, CSSA, and SSSA; 2015. p. 129-154. DOI: 10.2134/agronmonogr57.2013.0023

[29] Wang M, Yuan D, Zhang X. Genome Sequencing. In: Fang DD, Percy RG, editors. Cotton, 2nd ed., Agron. Monogr. 57. Madison: ASA, CSSA, and SSSA; 2015. p. 289-302. DOI: 10.2134/agronmonogr57.2013.0028

[30] Wu Z, Yang Y, Huang G, Lin J, Xia Y, Zhu Y. Cotton functional genomics reveals global insight into genome evolution and fiber development. Journal of Genetics and Genomics 2017;44(11):511-518. DOI: 10.1016/j.jgg.2017.09.009

[31] Li F, Fan G, Lu C, Xiao G, et al. Genome sequence of cultivated Upland cotton (*Gossypium hirsutum* TM-1) provides insights into genome evolution. Nature Biotechnology. 2015;33(5):524-530. DOI: 10.1038/nbt.3208

[32] Wang K, Huang G, Zhu Y. Transposable elements play an important role during cotton genome evolution and fiber cell development. Science China Life Sciences. 2016;59(2):112-121. DOI: 10.1007/s11427-015-4928-y

[33] Pan Y, Meng F, Wang X. Sequencing Multiple Cotton Genomes Reveals Complex Structures and Lays Foundation for Breeding. Front. Plant Sci. 2020;11:560096. DOI: 10.3389/fpls.2020.560096

[34] Orozco-Arias S, Isaza G, Guyot R. Retrotransposons in Plant Genomes: Structure, Identification, and Classification through Bioinformatics and Machine Learning. Int. J. Mol. Sci. 2019;20:3837. DOI: 10.3390/ijms20153837

[35] Palmer SA, Clapham AJ, Rose P, Freitas FO, et al. Archaeogenomic Evidence of Punctuated Genome Evolution in *Gossypium*. Mol. Biol. Evol. 2012;29(8):2031-2038. DOI: 10.1093/molbev/mss070

[36] Wang M, Li J, Wang P, Liu F, et al. Comparative Genome Analyses Highlight Transposon-Mediated Genome Expansion and the Evolutionary Architecture of 3D Genomic Folding in Cotton. Molecular Biology and Evolution. DOI: 10.1093/molbev/msab128

[37] Lu H, Cui X, Liu Z, Liu Y, et al. Discovery and annotation of a novel transposable element family in *Gossypium*. BMC Plant Biology. 2018;18(1):307. DOI: 10.1186/s12870-018-1519-7

[38] Wang M, Tu L, Yuan D, Zhu D, et al. Reference genome sequences of two cultivated allotetraploid cottons, *Gossypium hirsutum* and *Gossypium barbadense*. *Nat. Genet.* 2019;51:224-229. DOI: 10.1038/s41588-018-0282-x

[39] Page JT, Liechty ZS, Alexander RH, Clemons K, et al. DNA sequence evolution and rare homoeologous conversion in tetraploid cotton. PLoS Genet. 2016;12:e1006012. DOI: 10.1371/journal.pgen.1006012

[40] Zhang T, Hu Y, Jiang W, Fang L, et al. Sequencing of allotetraploid cotton (*Gossypium hirsutum* L. acc. TM-1) provides a resource for fiber improvement. *Nat. Biotechnol.* 2015;33:531-537. DOI: 10.1038/nbt.3207

[41] Yoo MJ, Wendel JF. Comparative evolutionary and developmental dynamics of the cotton (*Gossypium hirsutum*) fiber transcriptome. *PLoS Genet.* 2014;10:e1004073. DOI: 10.1371/journal.pgen.1004073

[42] Hu G, Koh J, Yoo MJ, Chen S, Wendel JF. Gene-Expression Novelty in Allopolyploid Cotton: A Proteomic Perspective. Genetics 2015;200:91-104. DOI: 10.1534/genetics.115.174367

[43] Hovav R, Faigenboim-Doron A, Kadmon N, Hu G, et al. A transcriptome profile for developing seed of polyploid cotton. The Plant Genome. 2015;8:eplantgenome2014.08.0041. DOI: 10.3835/plantgenome2014.08.0041

[44] Peng Z, Cheng H, Sun G, et al. Expression patterns and functional divergence of homologous genes accompanied by polyploidization in cotton (*Gossypium hirsutum* L.). Sci. China Life Sci. 2020;63:1565-1579. DOI: 10.1007/s11427-019-1618-7

[45] Fang L, Gong H, Hu Y, Liu C, et al. Genomic insights into divergence and dual domestication of cultivated

allotetraploid cottons. Genome Biology. 2017;18:33. DOI: 10.1186/s13059-017-1167-5

[46] Panchy N, Lehti-Shiu MD, Shiu SH. Evolution of gene duplication in plants. Plant Physiology. 2016;171:2294-2316. DOI: 10.1104/pp.16.00523

[47] Haigler CH, Betancur L, Stiff MR, Tuttle JR. Cotton fiber: a powerful single-cell model for cell wall and cellulose research. Front Plant Sci. 2012;3:104. DOI: 10.3389/fpls.2012.00104

[48] Yang Z, Qanmber G, Wang Z, Yang Z, Li F. Gossypium Genomics: Trends, Scope, and Utilization for Cotton Improvement. Trends Plant Sci. 2020;25:488-500. DOI: 10.1016/j.tplants.2019.12.011

[49] Snodgrass SJ, Jareczek J, Wendel JF. An examination of nucleotypic effects in diploid and polyploid cotton. AoB Plants. 2017;9:plw082. DOI: 10.1093/aobpla/plw082

[50] Brockington SF, Alvarez-Fernandez R, Landis JB, Alcorn K, et al. Evolutionary Analysis of the MIXTA Gene Family Highlights Potential Targets for the Study of Cellular Differentiation. Molecular Biology and Evolution. 2013;30:526-540. DOI: 10.1093/molbev/mss260

[51] Wu H, Tian Y, Wan Q, Fang L, et al. Genetics and evolution of MIXTA genes regulating cotton lint fiber development. New Phytol. 2018;217:883-895. DOI: 10.1111/nph.14844

[52] Zheng D, Ye W, Song Q, Han F, Zhang T, Chen ZJ. Histone Modifications Define Expression Bias of Homoeologous Genomes in Allotetraploid Cotton. Plant Physiol. 2016;172:1760-1771. DOI: 10.1104/pp.16.01210

[53] Gallagher JP, Grover CE, Hu G, Jareczek JJ, Wendel JF. Conservation and Divergence in Duplicated Fiber Coexpression Networks Accompanying Domestication of the Polyploid *Gossypium hirsutum* L. G3: Genes, Genomes, Genetics. 2020;10:2879-2892. DOI: 10.1534/g3.120.401362

[54] Ashraf J, Zuo D, Wang Q, Malik W, et al. Recent insights into cotton functional genomics: progress and future perspectives. Plant Biotechnology Journal. 2018;6:699-713. DOI: 10.1111/pbi.12856

[55] Fang L, Guan X, Zhang T. Asymmetric evolution and domestication in allotetraploid cotton (*Gossypium hirsutum* L.). The Crop Journal. 2017;5:159-165. DOI: 10.1016/j.cj.2016.07.001

[56] Xu Z, Yu JZ, Cho J, Yu J, Kohel RJ, Percy RG. Polyploidization Altered Gene Functions in Cotton (*Gossypium* spp.). PLoS ONE. 2010;5(12):e14351. DOI: 10.1371/journal.pone.0014351

[57] Zhu G, Li W, Wang G, Li L, Si Q, Cai C, Guo W. Genetic Basis of Fiber Improvement and Decreased Stress Tolerance in Cultivated Versus Semi-Domesticated Upland Cotton. Front. Plant Sci. 2019;10:1572. DOI: 10.3389/fpls.2019.01572

[58] Wendel JF, Cronn RC. Polyploidy and the evolutionary history of cotton. Adv Agron. 2003;78:139-186.

[59] Page JT, Huynh MD, Liechty ZS, Grupp K, et al. Insights into the Evolution of Cotton Diploids and Polyploids from Whole-Genome Re-sequencing. G3 (Bethesda). 2013;3(10):1809-18. DOI: 10.1534/g3.113.007229

[60] Buriev ZT, Saha S, Shermatov SE, Jenkins JN, et al. Molecular evolution of the clustered MIC-3 multigene family of

Gossypium species. Theor Appl Genet. 2011;123:1359-1373. DOI: 10.1007/s00122-011-1672-y

[61] Small RL, Wendel JF. Copy number lability and evolutionary dynamics of the Adh gene family in diploid and tetraploid cotton (*Gossypium*). Genetics. 2000;155:1913-1926.

[62] Small RL, Wendel JF. Differential evolutionary dynamics of duplicated paralogous Adh loci in allotetraploid cotton (*Gossypium*). Mol. Biol. Evol. 2002;19:597-607. DOI: 10.1093/oxfordjournals.molbev.a004119

Chapter 6

Soybean as a Model Crop to Study Plant Oil Genes: Mutations in FAD2 Gene Family

Sy M. Traore and Guohao He

Abstract

Plants have numerous fatty acid desaturase (FAD) enzymes regulating the unsaturation of fatty acids, which are encoded by a FAD gene family. The *FAD2* genes belong to such family and play a vital role in converting monounsaturated oleic acid to polyunsaturated linoleic acid. Oleic acid has the health benefits for humans, such as reduction in cholesterol level, antioxidation property, and industrial benefits like longer shelf life. The development of genotypes with high oleic acid content in seeds has become one of the primary goals in breeding oilseed plants. The identification and characterization of the *FAD2* genes in plants have been an important step to better manipulate gene expression to improve the seed oil quality. The induction of mutations in *FAD2* genes to reduce FAD2 enzyme activity has been an integral approach to generate genotypes with high oleic acid. This chapter will describe the FAD2 gene family in the model organism soybean and the correction of mutations in *FAD2* genes with the increase of oleic acid content. Leveraging advanced research of *FAD2* gene family in soybean promotes the study of *FAD2* genes in other legume species, including peanut. The future perspectives and challenges associated with mutations in *FAD2* genes will be discussed.

Keywords: legume, desaturase, genome editing, fatty acid, mutation, protein

1. Introduction

The legume family (Leguminosae) is the third-largest family of flowering plants, with over 800 genera and 20,000 species, after the Orchidaceae and Asteraceae [1]. It is classified into three sub-families: Papilionoideae, Caesalpinioideae, and Mimosoideae based on morphological characters [1]. The family presents incredibly diverse morphological characters, from giant rain forest trees and woody lianas, to desert shrubs, ephemeral herbs, herbaceous twining climbers, aquatics, and fire-adapted savanna species [1–3]. Two sub-families, Caesalpinioideae and Mimosoideae, are mostly woody trees and shrubs. Papilionoideae is the largest sub-family consisting of 476 genera and ~ 14,000 species, including most of the economically important legumes [4]. All papilionoids share a common ancestor and bear butterfly-shaped flowers [5, 6]. Within the Papilionoideae, there are four clades, phaseoloids, galegoids, genistoids, and dalbergoids, based on phylogenetic analyses [1, 4]. These clades cover the economically important food and feed legumes. For instance, the phaseoloid clade includes soybean, common bean, cowpea, and pigeon pea; the galegoid clade within the Hologalegina group includes medicago, chickpea, faba bean, lentil, and pea; the genistoid clade includes lupinus, and the dalbergoid clade includes peanut (**Figure 1**) [7, 8].

The pea (*Pisum sativum* L.) was the original model organism used in Mendel's discovery (1866) of the laws of inheritance, establishing the foundation of modern plant genetics [9, 10]. Although Mendel's peas were the first "model" plant, legume biology has long lagged behind more successful models from the Brassicaceae family or economically important cereals [10]. Due to legumes differing vastly in genome size, chromosome number, ploidy level, and reproductive biology, two legume species with smaller genome size in the Galegoid clade, *Medicago truncatula* and *Lotus japonicas*, were firstly selected as model organisms to demonstrate the referenced genetic system for legumes [11–13]. As the genome of soybean (*Glycine max* L.) has been available in 2010 [14], gene discovery in soybean is more efficient and feasible, providing a powerful high-throughput and non-targeted approach to gene expression and an excellent resource for comparative legume genomics. Although soybean has a relatively large genome compared with much smaller genomes of *Medicago* and *Lotus*, soybean is the most widely grown and economically important legume. Together with advantageous genome sequences, soybean is also considered as a model organism in legumes [15].

The existence of model organisms is fundamental for advancing genetic and genomic studies in crop species. Comprehensive biology study in the model organisms facilitates the transference of biological knowledge, gene function and expression, genomic information, and advanced tools to crop species. Fatty acids

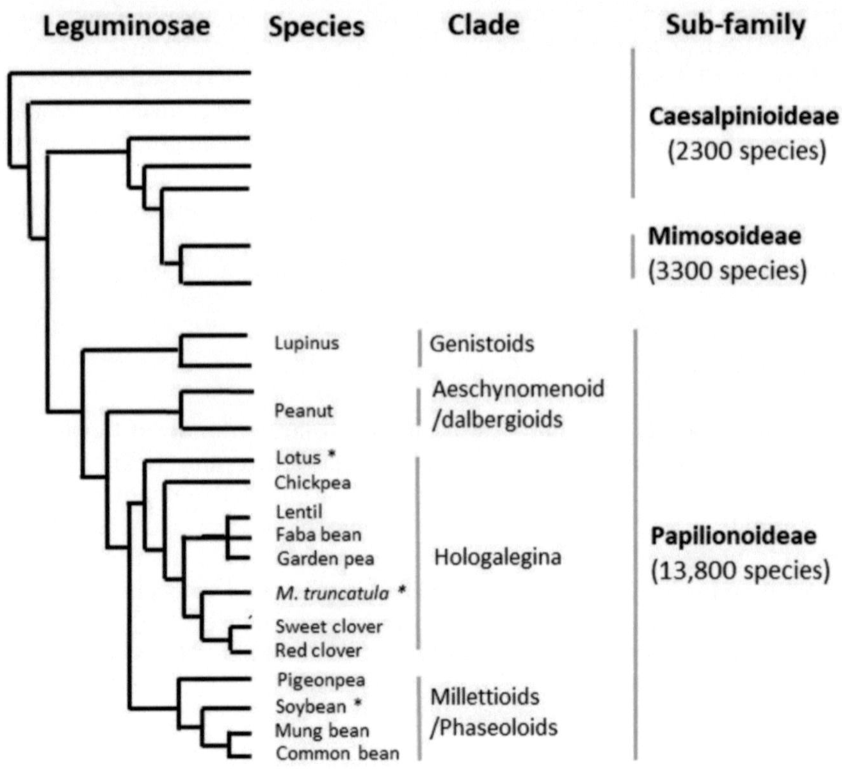

Figure 1.
*Phylogenetic relationships of sub-families, major clades within the sub-family Papilionoideae, and some economically important species in legumes (modified from references [7, 8]). *refer to model species.*

are essential components of cellular membranes, storage lipids, and precursors involved in plant metabolism and development [16]. The abundance of different fatty acids in plants is regulated by diverse fatty acid desaturases (FADs) enzymes [17]. Among FADs, the FAD2 enzyme converts monounsaturated oleic acid to polyunsaturated linoleic acid by adding a second double bond at the Δ12 position in the acyl chain. Manipulation of *FAD2* gene expression and enzyme activity in seeds enables the accumulation of oleic acids that benefit industries and consumers. This chapter aims to describe the FAD2 gene family in the model organism soybean. Mutations induced in *FAD2* genes and consequences from soybean to crop species, including peanut, are also discussed.

2. FAD gene family in the model organism soybean

Soybean seed oil is composed of approximately 20% of total seed composition, contributing the greatest concentrations of oil when compared to any food legume [18]. However, the concentration of oil is entirely dependent on the growing region, cultivar, and several environmental factors. As seeds develop, lipids, mostly triglycerides, are stored in cell oil bodies surrounding the larger protein bodies [19]. The fatty acid composition of most soybean seeds consists of 11% palmitic acid (16:0), 4% stearic acid (18:0), 25% oleic acid (18:1), 52% linoleic acid (18:2), and 8% linolenic acid (18,3) [20], with 24 other fatty acids in much lower quantities [21]. Synthesis of less common fatty acids occurs with similar structural configurations, which reside in cell membranes and storage lipids that are found in much lower quantities. This composition is mainly due to the physiological processes for seed dormancy and sustaining nutrition for young, recently germinated plants [18].

Fatty acids play an essential role in regulating the tolerance to various environmental stresses by altering the properties of cell membranes [22, 23]. During the desaturation of fatty acid in plant cells, the number and position of the double bonds in a fatty acid chain influence its physical and physiological properties [24, 25], the membranes function, and the proper growth and development [24]. The release of the genomic sequence has allowed the identification of *FAD* genes firstly in Arabidopsis followed by many crop species, including oilseed crops, such as soybean [26, 27], cotton [28, 29], cacao [30], peanut, and olive [31, 32]. Different fatty acid desaturases (FADs) are involved in the desaturation of fatty acids, including the microsomal Δ12 desaturase (FAD2), the microsomal ω3 desaturase (FAD3), the trans ω3 desaturase (FAD4), the Δ7 desaturase (FAD5), the plastidial Δ12 desaturase (FAD6), the plastidial ω3 desaturase (FAD7), and the plastidial ω3 desaturase (FAD8) [33]. Among these desaturases, FAD2 and FAD6 are ω6 desaturases that convert monounsaturated fatty acid (oleic acid) to polyunsaturated fatty acid (linoleic acid) in the endoplasmic reticulum (ER) and plastids, respectively. FAD3, FAD7, and FAD8 are ω3 desaturases that synthesize linolenic from linoleic acid in the ER (FAD3) and plastids (FAD7 and FAD8) (**Figure 2**) [34, 35]. FAD4 and FAD5 specifically produce monounsaturated acid from palmitic acid for phosphatidylglycerol (PG) and monogalactosyldiacylglycerol (MGDG), respectively [36]. The content of oleic and linoleic acids affects the oxidative stability and nutritional value of edible oil [37]. Linoleic acid is a polyunsaturated fatty acid that plays a vital role in human health and nutrition; however, it has the disadvantage of decreasing the stability, flavor, and shelf life of the edible oil [38, 39]. Conversely, the oil higher in oleic acid has advantages of higher oxidative stability and long shelf life [40], increase structural integrity at a higher cooking temperature [41], and nutrition benefits to reduce low-density lipoprotein (LDL) cholesterol [42], suppress tumor formation, and protect from inflammatory diseases [43]. Therefore, human

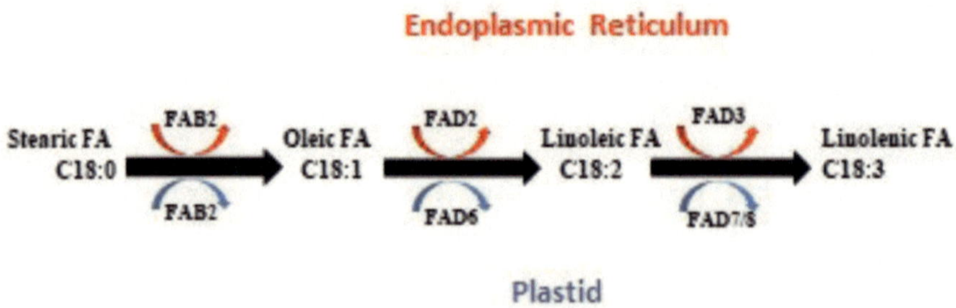

Figure 2.
Illustration of a part of the fatty acid biosynthesis pathway.

Gene	Accession number	Chromosome	References
GmFAD2–1A	Glyma.10G278000	10	[47, 50, 51]
GmFAD2–1B	Glyma.20G111000	20	[47, 50, 51]
GmFAD2–2A	Glyma.19G147300	19	[47, 50, 51]
GmFAD2–2B	Glyma.19G147400	19	[47, 50, 51]
GmFAD2–2C	Glyma.03G144500	03	[47, 50, 51]
GmFAD2–2D	Glyma.09G111900	09	[52]
GmFAD2–2E	Glyma.15G195200	15	[52]

Table 1.
List of FAD2 genes in soybean.

consumption of soybean seed oil demands higher oleic acid and lower linoleic acid. Efforts have been made to identify *FAD2* genes that significantly affect fatty acid biosynthesis, to understand their inheritance, and to manipulate gene expression to develop oilseed crops with high content of oleic acid [44–49].

2.1 *FAD2* gene family in soybean

In soybean, the *FAD* gene has two copies, *GmFAD2–1* and *GmFAD2–2*, each of them has two members (*GmFAD2–1A* and *GmFAD2–1B*) and three members (*GmFAD2–2A*, *GmFAD2–2B*, and *GmFAD2–2C*), respectively [47, 50, 51]. Using both soybase and phytozome databases, an additional two novel *FAD2–2* members, named *GmFAD2–2D* and *GmFAD2–2E*, were identified (**Table 1**) [52]. Among the identified *FAD* genes in soybean, the FAD2–1A and FAD2–1B EST analysis suggested that the *GmFAD2–1A* and *GmFAD2–1B* are actively expressed in developing seeds and constitute the seed specific paralogs in the soybean genome [53]. *GmFAD2–2A* possessed a deletion of 100 bp in the coding region and therefore was predicted to be non-functional [50]. *GmFAD2–2B* and *GmFAD2–2C* were found to display ubiquitous expression in all the vegetative tissues of the soybean plant, *GmFAD2–2D* was expressed in the flower, seed, and nodule, while *GmFAD2–2E* expression was exclusively confined to the pod and seed with a low level of expression.

Because of nutritional and health value, soybean breeders have been paying special attention to screen for the source of high oleic acid in soybean germplasm. Two mid-oleic acid mutant lines carrying a mutant allele *GmFAD2–1a* were identified from phenotype-based screening [54]. Through Targeting Induced Local Lesions In Genomes (TILLING), another mutant *GmFAD2–1b* was found. When combining mutant *GmFAD2–1a* and *GmFAD2–1b* alleles into one line, oleic acid content was increased to 83%. Similarly, a total of 22 plant introductions (PIs) were screened for high oleic acid content in soybean seeds [50]. Two genotypes, PI 603452 and PI 2833270, were identified with increased oleic acid. Sequence analysis showed mutations occurred in the *FAD2–1A* gene of PI 603452 and in the *FAD2–1B* gene of PI 283327, respectively. When PI 603452 was crossed with PI 283327, a soybean line carrying both homozygous *FAD2–1A* and *FAD2–1B* mutants was found in the following segregation generations. Fatty acid content analysis showed that oleic acid content increased up to 82–86%, and the level of linoleic and linolenic acids was reduced, while only 20% of oleic acid in wild type soybean lines. Further mutation analysis using (TILLING) by sequencing also demonstrated that mutations within *GmFAD2–1A* and *GmFAD2–1B* affect seed oleic acid content in soybean [52]. These two genes have played an important role in converting oleic acid to linoleic acid and directly determining the composition of oleic acid in soybean seeds. *FAD2* gene is 1,164 bp long with an open reading frame coding for about 387 amino acids [55]. It contains two exons and a single large intron that is embedded within the 5′-untranslated region (5' UTR) and has a promoter function to regulate the expression level of *FAD2* [56, 57]. In soybean, *GmFAD2–1A* and *GmFAD2–1B* share 99% coding sequence identity and are located in paralogous regions of chromosomes 10 and 20, respectively [58].

2.2 Mutations in *FAD2* genes

Natural mutations in both GmFAD2–1A and GmFAD2–1B in soybean led to a high level of oleic acid, indicating that mutations in both genes can suppress *FAD2* gene expression to loss of enzyme function resulted in accumulation of oleic acid and decrease in linoleic acid content. Consequently, mutations induced in both genes become a critical step to improve seed oil. Various mutagenesis tools are used to target these two genes in the coding region or promoter region. A previous study showed that RNAi silencing reduced *GmFAD2* expression and increased oleic acid from 20% to greater than 80% [59]. Transcription activator-like effector nucleases (TALENs) technique was used to target and cleave conserved DNA sequences in both genes *FAD2–1A* and *FAD2–1B* [60]. In four of 19 transgenic soybean lines expressing the TALENs, FAD2–1A and FAD2–1B mutations were observed in the DNA extracted from leaf tissues, and three of the four lines transmitted heritable FAD2–1 mutations to the next generation. The fatty acid profile of the seed was dramatically changed in plants with homozygous mutations in both *FAD2–1A* and *FAD2–1B*, resulting in oleic acid increasing from 20% to 80% and linoleic acid decreased from 50% to under 4% [60]. The chemical mutagen (EMS) was used in the germplasm to generate mutant lines with high oleic acid content [61]. Sequence analysis revealed lines with mutation on the *FAD2–1A* and *FAD2–1B*. Further crossing of the single mutant lines released the *FAD2–1a* and *FAD2–1b* double mutant with high oleic acid content. Biological mutagens have also been used to induce mutations in *FAD2* gene to develop high oleic acid lines.

In recent years, the RNA-guided CRISPR/Cas9 system has appeared as a promising tool in site-directed mutagenesis. The release of the genomic sequence of soybean and the characterization of the FAD2 allow to precisely induce mutations on the coding sequence of these *FAD2* genes. Kim et al. [62] first used CRISPR/Cpf1 system in soybean and successfully induced deletion mutations in *FAD2* genes though edited plants were not available (**Figure 3**). The CRISPR/Cas9 system was also used to target the soybean *FAD2* genes. Expression and sequence analysis confirmed the alteration of the target genes was corrected with high oleic acid up to 65.58% while low linoleic acid to 16.08% [48]. CRISPR/Cas9 technology

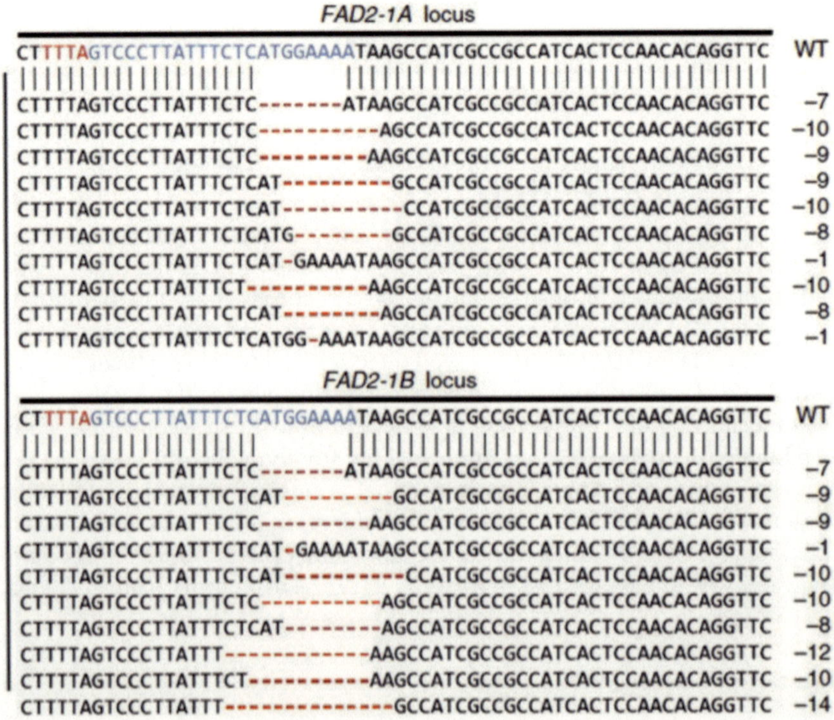

Figure 3.
Demonstration of deletion mutations identified at the target site (blue) of FAD2 genes using CRISPR/Cpf1 (cited from Kim et al. [62]).

induced homozygous mutations in *GmFAD2–1A* alone generated high oleic acid without adverse effects on plant development [63]. Two gRNAs simultaneously targeting two sites within the second exons of both *GmFAD2–1A* and *GmFAD2–1B* showed dramatic increases in oleic acid content to over 80%, whereas linoleic acid decreased to 1.3–1.7% [56]. Transgene-free high oleic homozygous genotypes could be obtained through segregation generations, in their case, as early as the T1 generation. A gRNA was designed to target the coding region in the first exon of *GmFAD2–1A* and *GmFAD2–2A*, resulting in the oleic acid content increased from 17.1% to 73.5%, and the linoleic acid content decreased from 62.9% to 12.2% [49]. The coding region of *FAD2* gene contains four transmembrane domains and three histidine boxes (H-box) in soybean (**Figure 4**) [53]. The histidine residues are essential for the catalytic function of the FAD2 enzyme; substituting histidine with a different amino acid disrupts its desaturase function [64]. High efficiency of mutagenesis using CRISPR-based gene editing provides a promising tool to induce mutations within the sequence of *FAD2* genes. With intensive efforts, high oleic acid varieties, Vistiv Gold and Plenish, were developed by Monsanto and DuPont companies, respectively [49].

In addition to alter the coding region, mutations in the promoter and intron can influence *FAD2* gene expression. The *FAD2* intron has promoter activity because it harbors promoter-like sequence structures, including TATA and CAAT boxes, as well as many potential *cis*-elements [56]. Bioinformatics analyses of *FAD2* intron revealed the CGATT motif and the 5' UTR Py-rich stretch motif that enhanced gene expression [65]. Mutations in the TATA-box of the promoter reduced the promoter's function [66]. Therefore, mutations induced in both intron and promoter can manipulate the gene expression of *FAD2*, though few studies focus on this aspect in soybean.

```
                                                                        TM-1
A   MGLAKETTMGGRGRVAKVEVQGKKPLSRVPNTKPPFTVGQLKKAIPPHCFQRSLLTSFSY
B   MGLAKET IMGGGGRVAKVE I QQKKPLSRVPNTKPPFTVGQLKKAIPPHCFQRSLLTSLSY      60

                                       TM-2                 H-box I
A   VVYDLSFAFIFYIATTYFHLLPQPFSLIAWP IYWVLQGCLLTGVWV IAHECGHHAFSKYQ     120
B   VVYDLSLAFIFYIATTYFHLLPHPFSLIAWP IYWVLQGC ILTGVWV IAHECGHHAFSKYP    120

                               H-box II
A   WVDDVVGLTLHSTLLVPYFSWK ISHRRHHSNTGSLDRDEVFVPKPKSKVAWFSKYLNNPL      180
B   WVDDVMGLTVHSTLLVPYFSWKISHRRHHSNTGSLDRDEVFVPKPKSKVAWYTKYLNNPL       180

                                                                  TM-3
A   GRAVSLLVTLTIGWPMYLAFNVSGRPYDSFASHYHPYAPIYSNRERLLIYVSDVALFSVT       240
B   GRAASLL I TLTIGWPLYLAFNVSGRPYDGFASHYHPYAPIYSNRERLLIYVSDVALFSVT     240

                      TM-4
A   YSLYRVAT LKGLVWLLCVYGVPLLIVNGFLVTITYLQHTHFALPHYDSSEWDWLKGALAT      300
B   YLLYRVATMKGLVWLLCVYGVPLLIVNGFLVTITYLQHTHYALPHYDSSEWDWLRGALAT       300

                      H-box III
A   MDRDYGILNKVFHHITDTHVAHHLFSTMPHYHAMEATNA IKPILGEYYQFDDTPFYKALW      360
B   MDRDYGILNKVFHHITDTHVAHHLFSTMPHYHA TEATNAMKPILGEYYRFDDTPFYKALW      360

A   REARECLYVEPDEGTSEKGVYWYRNKY              387
B   REARECLYVEPDEGTSEKGVYWYRNKY              387
```

Figure 4.
Alignment of FAD2–1A and FAD2–1B amino acid sequences. The difference in Amino acids between A and B is highlighted in red. There are four transmembrane domains and three H-box in the coding region of FAD2 enzyme in soybean (modified from Tang et al. [53]).

2.3 *FAD2* genes from model organism soybean to crop species peanut

Peanut (*A. hypogaea* L.) is an economically important oilseed crop like soybean but belongs to a different clade from soybean. Comparison of *FAD2* genes in peanut and soybean, peanut has an open reading frame without intron but one intron in soybean. Compared to soybean, peanut seed has a higher content of oleic acid (36–67%) and a lower level of linoleic acid (15–43%) [67]. The first natural mutant peanut genotype with 80% of oleic acid content and 2% of linoleic acid in seeds was reported in 1987 [68]. Research studies have demonstrated that the natural mutant genotype with high oleic acid was associated with mutations in the *FAD2* genes. Two homeologous *AhFAD2A* and *AhFAD2B* genes are responsible for converting oleic acid to linoleic acid, located on the chromosomes 9 and 19 of the A and B genomes in the allotetraploidy peanut, respectively [69, 70]. The coding region of both genes has a length of 1,140 base pairs (bp) with 99% sequence homology and only 11 bp differences. The comparison between the high oleic acid line (F435) and the low oleic acid line (Tampson 90) revealed the presence of two mutations on the coding sequence of *AhFAD2*. The first mutation was a substitution of base guanine (G) to the base adenine (A) at the 448 bp position from the start codon in *AhFAD2A*, resulting in a missense amino acid from aspartic acid to asparagine. The second mutation was an insertion of the purine base adenine (A) at 441–442 bp position in *AhFAD2B*, leading to the shift in the amino acid reading frame, consequently generating premature stop codon [70]. Both spontaneous mutations that occurred on *AhFAD2A* and *AhFAD2B* alleles led to 80% of oleic acid and 2% linoleic acid [71]. After screening the Chinese mini core collection, 53.1% of genotypes carrying natural mutation G448A in the *AhFAD2A* gene and 46.9% with no mutations were observed [72]. Interestingly, 82.8% of this mutation existed in *A. hypogaea* subsp. *hypogaea* while 15.4% was observed in *A. hypogaea* subsp. *fastigiat*. In addition, no mutations were detected in the

AhFAD2B gene alone in any lines of the collection. Over 4000 peanut genotypes were screened, and two natural mutant lines PI 342664 and PI 342666 with high oleic acid, were identified [73]. In these two natural mutant lines, sequencing results of the coding region showed the same substitution of G448A in *AhFAD2A*, but a different substitution of C301G in *AhFAD2B*, resulting in an amino acid substitution of H101D. These reports demonstrated that mutations occurred in the coding region in either one or both of *AhFAD2A* and *AhFAD2B* genes alter enzymatic activity that leads to the higher oleate trait in mutant genotypes [73]. In addition to the natural *FAD2* mutations in peanut, various chemical and physical mutagens, for example, X rays, EMS, gamma rays, and sodium azide, were used to generate mutations in *FAD2* genes to increase oleic acid content in seeds. However, these methods generated many other mutations in the genome other than in the target gene [74–77]. Yuan et al. [78] was the first use of CRISPR/Cas9 technology in peanut to induce mutations in *FAD2* genes. The result showed that the same mutations of *AhFAD2* genes that occurred in nature could be induced by gene editing. We have increased oleic acid content with different levels using a CRISPR-based gene editing approach targeting several locations in the coding region and *cis*-regulatory RY element (CATGCATG) and 2S seed protein motif (CAAACAC) in the promoter region of peanut. Inducement of mutations in both coding and promoter regions using the CRISPR-based gene editing technology is ongoing in our peanut research. Hopefully, through gene editing, genotypes with high oleic acid content in soybean and peanut will be developed to complement the conventional breeding method.

3. Future perspectives and challenges in the mutagenesis of *FAD2* genes

As a model organism and economically important species in legumes, soybean has been intensively investigated in genetics and genomics for its genetic improvement. Precision gene editing systems have been used to change the profile of the soybean seed fatty acid panel. The TALEN technology has been used to target the *FAD2* genes, and induced mutations materialize by a significant increase of the oleic fatty acid content. CRISPR-based gene editing system has advantages of ease use, accuracy, high efficiency, and success in a wide range of crop species to induce mutations in *FAD2* genes. Transgene-free genotypes can be obtained through recombination of edited plants in the following segregation generations. However, the application of CRISPR-based gene editing is a challenge in polyploidy species due to multiple copies of target genes. Different mutant allele combinations would also change the content of oleic acid. Moreover, a complete loss of FAD2 function could result in important development defects due to the lack of polyunsaturated fatty acids that play a crucial role in maintaining the fluidity of the cell membrane in a cold temperature environment. The better strategy to accumulate oleic acid in seed only may implement gene editing to target cis-regulatory elements that implicate seed-specific gene expression in the promoter and avoid knocking down FAD2 expression in the entire plant.

Genetic transformation methods were developed using particle bombardment meristem cells and shoot tips and somatic embryogenesis in soybean. The establishment of these technologies has permitted the generation of soybean lines to improve its oil quality. However, legume species are generally difficult to transform and regenerate. The tissue culture procedure is time-consuming, genotype dependent, and recalcitrant to regenerate adventitious shoots from explants, particularly in soybean and peanut. Methodology to avoid tissue culture should be developed, such as floral dipping for Agrobacterium mediate delivery.

4. Conclusions

Fatty acids are essential components of cellular membranes and storage lipids that are regulated in part through the action of fatty acid desaturases (FADs) and related enzymes. *FAD2* gene encoding fatty acid desaturase 2 enzyme is responsible for converting oleic acid to linoleic acid in the developing seeds and directly affects seed oil quality in oilseed crops. Intensive genetic and genomic studies of *FAD2* genes in soybean as a model organism provide valuable information on understanding FAD2 gene family members to other oilseed crops. Due to high oleic acid's nutritional and health value, efforts have been focused on generating mutations in the *FAD2* gene, which could lead to high oleic acid content. Mutations that occurred in both *FAD2–1A* and *FAD2–1B* genes in soybean can result in the highest oleic acid content. Among the tools used for mutagenesis, CRISPR/Cas9 technology is a promising approach to target multiple genes simultaneously and precisely to efficiently induce mutations.

Acknowledgements

The authors would like to thank the financial support from USDA/NIFA (2018-67014-27572).

Author details

Sy M. Traore and Guohao He*
Tuskegee University, Tuskegee, USA

*Address all correspondence to: ghe@tuskegee.edu

References

[1] Lewis G, Schrire B, Mackinder B, Lock M (eds). Legumes of the world. Royal Botanic Gardens, Kew, UK. 2005.

[2] Doyle JJ, Luckow MA. The rest of the iceberg. Legume diversity and evolution in a phylogenetic context. Plant Physiol. 2003;131:900-910.

[3] Bruneau A, Doyle JJ, Herendeen P, et al. Legume phylogeny and classification in the 21st century: Progress, prospects and lessons for other species–rich clades. TAXON. 2013;62:217-248.

[4] Smỳkal P, Coyne CJ, Ambrose MJ, et al. Legume crops phylogeny and genetic diversity for science and breeding. Crit Rev Plant Sci. 2015;34:43-104.

[5] Doyle JJ. DNA data and legume phylogeny: a progress report. In: Advances in Legume Systematics. Pp. 11-30. Part 7: Phylogeny. Crisp M, Doyle JJ. Eds. Royal Botanic Gardens, Kew, UK. 1995

[6] Lavin M, Herendeen PS, Wojciechowski MF. Evolutionary rates analysis of Leguminosae implicates a rapid diversification of lineages during the tertiary. Syst Biol. 2005;54:575-594.

[7] Choi HK, Mun JH, Kim DJ, Zhu HY, Baek JM, Mudge J, Roe B, Ellis N, Doyle J, Kiss GB, Young ND, Cook DR. Estimating genome conservation between crop and model legume species. PNAS. 2004;101(43): 15289-15294

[8] Gepts P, Beavis WD, Brummer EC, et al. Legumes as a model plant family. Genomics for food and feed report of the cross-legume advances through genomics conference. Plant Physiol. 2005;137:1228-1235.

[9] Smýkal P, Vernoud V, Blair MW, et al. The role of the testa during development and in establishment of dormancy of the legume seed. Front Plant Sci. 2014;DOI:10.3389/fpls.2014.00351.

[10] Smykal P, von Wettberg EJB, McPhee KM. Legume genetics and biology: from Mendel's pea to legume genomics. Int J Mol Sci. 2020;21:3336, doi: 10.3390/ijms21093336

[11] Barker DG, Bianchi S, Blondon F, et al. Medicago truncatula, a model plant for studying the molecular genetics of the Rhizobium-legume symbiosis. Plant Mol Biol Report. 1990;8:40-49.

[12] Cook DR. Medicago truncatula-a model in the making! Curr Opin Plant Biol. 1999;2:301-304.

[13] Sato S, Nakamura Y, Kaneko T, et al. Genome structure of the legume, *Lotus japonicus*. DNA Res. 2008;15:227-239.

[14] Schmutz J, Canon SB, Schlueter J, Ma JX, Mitros T, Nelson W, et al. Genome sequence of the palaeopolyploid soybean. Nature. 2010;463:178-183.

[15] Ferguson BJ, Gresshoff PM. Soybean as a model legume. In: Grain Legumes, Species issue on Model Legumes. 2009;7

[16] Ohlrogge J, Browse J. Lipid biosynthesis. Plant Cell. 1995;7:957.

[17] Lee MW, Padilla CS, Gupta C, Galla A, Pereira A, Li JM, Goggin FL. The fatty acid desaturase2 family in tomato contributes to primary metabolism and stress responses. Plant Physiology. 2020;182:1083-1099

[18] Bewley JD, Bradford KJ, Hilhorst HW, et al. Structure and composition. In: *Seeds*. Springer, 2013, pp. 1-25.

[19] Lee KR, Kim SH, Go YS, Jung SM, Roh KH, Kim JB, Suh MC, Lee S, Kim HU. Molecular cloning and

functional analysis of two *FAD2* genes from American grape (Vitis labrusca L.). Gene. 2012;509(2):189-194.

[20] Fehr WR. Breeding for modified fatty acid composition in soybean. Crop Sci. 2007;47:S-72.

[21] Wilson RF. Seed composition. Soybeans Improv Prod Uses. 2004;16:621-677.

[22] Kachroo A, Kachroo P. Fatty acid–derived signals in plant defense. Annu Rev Phytopathol. 2009;47:153-176.

[23] Iba K. Acclimative response to temperature stress in higher plants: approaches of gene engineering for temperature tolerance. Annu Rev Plant Biol. 2002;53:225-245.

[24] Shanklin J, Cahoon EB. Desaturation and related modifications of fatty acids. Annu Rev Plant Biol. 1998;49:611-641.

[25] Wu Q, Liu T, Liu H, Zheng GC. Unsaturated fatty acid: metabolism, synthesis and gene regulation. Afr J Biotechnol. 2009;8(9):1782-1785.

[26] Chi Y, Huang F, Liu H, et al. An APETALA1-like gene of soybean regulates flowering time and specifies floral organs. J Plant Physiol. 2011;168:2251-2259.

[27] Román Á, Andreu V, Hernández ML, et al. Contribution of the different omega-3 fatty acid desaturase genes to the cold response in soybean. J Exp Bot. 2012;63:4973-4982.

[28] Yurchenko OP, Park S, Ilut DC, et al. Genome-wide analysis of the omega-3 fatty acid desaturase gene family in Gossypium. BMC Plant Biol. 2014;14:1-15.

[29] Liu G, Mei H, Wang S, et al. Association mapping of seed oil and protein contents in upland cotton. Euphytica. 2015;205:637-645.

[30] Zhang Y, Maximova SN, Guiltinan MJ. Characterization of a stearoyl-acyl carrier protein desaturase gene family from chocolate tree, *Theobroma cacao* L. Front Plant Sci. 2015;6:239.

[31] Banilas G, Nikiforiadis A, Makariti I, et al. Discrete roles of a microsomal linoleate desaturase gene in olive identified by spatiotemporal transcriptional analysis. Tree Physiol. 2007;27:481-490.

[32] Hernández ML, Sicardo MD, Martínez-Rivas JM. Differential contribution of endoplasmic reticulum and chloroplast ω-3 fatty acid desaturase genes to the linolenic acid content of olive (*Olea europaea*) fruit. Plant Cell Physiol. 2016;57:138-151.

[33] Wallis JG, Browse J. Mutants of Arabidopsis reveal many roles for membrane lipids. Prog Lipid Res. 2002;41:254-278.

[34] Gibson S, Arondel V, Iba K, et al. Cloning of a temperature-regulated gene encoding a chloroplast [omega]-3 desaturase from *Arabidopsis thaliana*. Plant Physiol. 1994;106:1615-1621.

[35] Berberich T, Harada M, Sugawara K, et al. Two maize genes encoding ω-3 fatty acid desaturase and their differential expression to temperature. Plant Mol Biol. 1998;36:297-306.

[36] Murphy DJ, Piffanelli P. Fatty acid desaturases: structure, mechanism and regulation. Plant lipid biosynthesis. 1998;1:95-130.

[37] Cao Y, Wang W, Xu Y, et al. Enzymatic synthesis of extremely pure triacylglycerols enriched in conjugated linoleic acids. Molecules. 2013;18: 9704-9716.

[38] Guan L-L, Wang Y-B, Shen H, et al. Molecular Cloning and Expression Analysis of Genes Encoding Two

Microsomal Oleate Desaturases (FAD2) from Safflower (*Carthamus tinctorius* L.). Plant Mol Biol Report. 2012;30:139-148.

[39] Pandey MK, Wang ML, Qiao L, et al. Identification of QTLs associated with oil content and mapping FAD2 genes and their relative contribution to oil quality in peanut (*Arachis hypogaea* L.). BMC Genet. 2014;15:133.

[40] Ge Y, Chang Y, Xu W, et al. Sequence variations in the *FAD2* gene in seeded pumpkins. Genet Mol Res. 2015;14:17482-17488.

[41] Warner K, Orr P, Parrott L, et al. Effects of frying oil composition on potato chip stability. J Am Oil Chem Soc. 1994;71:1117-1121.

[42] Mattson FH, Grundy SM. Comparison of effects of dietary saturated, monounsaturated, and polyunsaturated fatty acids on plasma lipids and lipoproteins in man. J Lipid Res. 1985;26:194-202.

[43] Yamaki T, Nagamine I, Fukumoto K, et al. High oleic peanut oil modulates promotion stage in lung tumorigenesis of mice treated with methyl nitrosourea. Food Sci Technol Res. 2005;11:231-235.

[44] Shah S, Xin Z, Browse J. Overexpression of the FAD3 desaturase gene in a mutant of Arabidopsis. Plant Physiol. 1997;114:1533-1539.

[45] Matsuda H, Kageura T, Oda M, et al. Effects of constituents from the bark of *Magnolia obovata* on nitric oxide production in lipopolysaccharide-activated macrophages. Chem Pharm Bull (Tokyo). 2001;49:716-720.

[46] Bilyeu KD, Palavalli L, Sleper DA, et al. Three microsomal omega-3 fatty-acid desaturase genes contribute to soybean linolenic acid levels. Crop Sci. 2003;43:1833-1838.

[47] Schlueter JA, Vasylenko-Sanders IF, Deshpande S, et al. The FAD2 gene family of soybean: Insights into the structural and functional divergence of a paleopolyploid genome. Crop Sci. 2007;47:S-14-S-26.

[48] Amin MZ, Islam T, Mostofa F, et al. Comparative assessment of the physicochemical and biochemical properties of native and hybrid varieties of pumpkin seed and seed oil (*Cucurbita maxima* Linn.). Heliyon. 2019; 5: e02994.

[49] Wu G, Shen Y, Nie R, et al. The bioactive compounds and cellular antioxidant activity of Herbaceous peony (Paeonia lactiflora Pall) seed oil from China. J Food Sci. 2020;85: 3815-3822.

[50] Pham A-T, Lee J-D, Shannon JG, et al. Mutant alleles of *FAD2-1A* and *FAD2-1B* combine to produce soybeans with the high oleic acid seed oil trait. BMC Plant Biol. 2010;10:195.

[51] Zhang L, Yang X, Zhang Y, et al. Changes in oleic acid content of transgenic soybeans by antisense RNA mediated posttranscriptional gene silencing. Int J Genomics. 2014;2014: e921950.

[52] Lakhssassi N, Zhou Z, Liu S, et al. Characterization of the *FAD2* Gene family in soybean reveals the limitations of gel-based TILLING in genes with high copy number. Front Plant Sci. 2017;DOI: 10.3389/fpls.2017.00324.

[53] Tang GQ, Novitzky WP, Griffin HC, Huber SC, Dewey RE. Oleate desaturase enzymes of soybean: evidence of regulation through differential stability and phosphorylation. The Plant J. 2005;44:433-446.

[54] Hoshino T, Takagi Y, Anai T. Novel *GmFAD2-1b* mutant alleles created by reverse genetics induce marked elevation of oleic acid content in

soybean seeds in combination with *GmFAD2-1a* mutant alleles. Breeding Sci. 2010;60:419-425.

[55] Dar AA, Choudhury AR, Kancharla PK, et al. The *FAD2* Gene in plants: occurrence, regulation, and role. Front Plant Sci. 2017;8:1789.

[56] Xiao G, Zhang ZQ, Yin CF, Liu RY, Wu XM, Tan TL Chen SY, Lu CM, Guan CY. Characterization of the promoter and 5'-UTR intron of oleic acid desaturase (FAD2) gene in *Brassica napus*. Gene. 2014;545:45-55.

[57] Zeng FQ, Roslinsky V, Cheng BF. Mutations in the promoter, intron and CDC of two *FAD2* generate multiple alleles modulating linoleic acid level in yellow mustard. Scientific Report. 2017;7:8284.

[58] Do PT, Nguyen CX, Bui HT, et al. Demonstration of highly efficient dual gRNA CRISPR/Cas9 editing of the homeologous *GmFAD2-1A* and *GmFAD2-1B* genes to yield a high oleic, low linoleic and α-linolenic acid phenotype in soybean. BMC Plant Biol. 2019;19:311.

[59] Mroczka A, Roberts PD, Fillatti JJ, et al. An intron sense suppression construct targeting soybean FAD2-1 requires a double-stranded RNA-producing inverted repeat T-DNA insert. Plant Physiol. 2010;153:882-891.

[60] Haun W, Coffman A, Clasen BM, et al. Improved soybean oil quality by targeted mutagenesis of the fatty acid desaturase 2 gene family. *Plant* Biotechnol J. 2014;12:934-940.

[61] Combs R, Bilyeu K. Novel alleles of FAD2-1A induce high levels of oleic acid in soybean oil. Mol Breed. 2019;39:79.

[62] Kim M, Schultz S, Nelson RL, et al. Identification and fine mapping of a soybean seed protein QTL from PI 407788A on chromosome 15. Crop Sci. 2016;56:219-225.

[63] Hou ZH, Wu Y, Cheng Q, Dong LD, Lu SJ, Nan HY, Gan ZR, Liu BH. Creation of high oleic acid soybean mutation plant by CRISPR/Cas9. Acta Agronomica Sinica. 2019;45(6):839-847.

[64] Shanklin J, Whittle E, Fox BG. Eight histidine residues are catalytically essential in a membrane-associated iron enzyme, stearoyl-CoA desaturase, and are conserved in alkane hydroxylase and xylene monooxygenase. Biochemistry. 1994;33:12787-12794.

[65] Parra G, Bradnam K, Rose AB, Korf I. Comparative and functional analysis of intron-mediated enhancement signals reveals conserved features among plants. Nucleic Acids Research. 2011;39:5328-5337.

[66] Zeng FQ, Roslinsky V, Cheng BF. Mutations in the promoter, intron and CDC of two *FAD2* generate multiple alleles modulating linoleic acid level in yellow mustard. Scientific Report. 2017;7:8284.

[67] Moore KM, Knauft DA. The Inheritance of high oleic acid in peanut. J Hered. 1989;80:252-253.

[68] Norden AJ, Gorbet DW, Knauft DA, et al. Variability in oil quality among peanut genotypes in the Florida Breeding Program1. Peanut Sci. 1987;14:7-11.

[69] Jung S, Swift D, Sengoku E, et al. The high oleate trait in the cultivated peanut [Arachis hypogaea L.]. I. Isolation and characterization of two genes encoding microsomal oleoyl-PC desaturases. Mol Gen Genet MGG. 2000;263:796-805.

[70] Chu Y, Holbrook CC, Ozias-Akins P. Two alleles of *ahFAD2B* control the high oleic acid trait in cultivated peanut. Crop Sci. 2009;49:2029-2036.

[71] López Y, Nadaf HL, Smith OD, et al. Isolation and characterization of the

Δ12-fatty acid desaturase in peanut (*Arachis hypogaea* L.) and search for polymorphisms for the high oleate trait in Spanish market-type lines. Theor Appl Genet. 2000;101:1131-1138.

[72] Lei Y, Jiang HF, Wen QG, Huang JQ, Yan LY, Liao BS. Frequencies of *ahFAD2A* alleles in Chinese peanut mini core collection and its correlation with oleic acid content. Acta Agron Sin. 2010;36(11):1864-1869.

[73] Wang ML, Tonnis B, Charles YQ, Pinnow D, Tishchenko V, Pederson GA. Newly identified natural high-oleate mutant from *Arachis hypogaea* L. subsp *hypogaea*. Mol Breed. 2015;35:186.

[74] Sharma ND, Santha IM, Patil SH, et al. Fatty acid and amino acid composition of groundnut mutants. Plant Foods Hum Nutr. 1985;35:3-8.

[75] Dwivedi SL, Nigam SN, Prasad MVR. Induced genetic variation for seed quality traits in groundnut. Int Arachis Newsl. 1998;18:44-46.

[76] Badigannavar AM, Murty GSS. Genetic enhancement of groundnut through gamma ray induced mutagenesis, http://inis.iaea.org/Search/search.aspx?orig_q=RN:39030970 (2007, accessed 22 July 2021).

[77] Mondal S, Badigannavar AM, D'Souza SF. Induced variability for fatty acid profile and molecular characterization of high oleate mutant in cultivated groundnut (*Arachis hypogaea* L.). Plant Breed. 2011;130:242-247.

[78] Yuan M, Zhu J, Gong L, et al. Mutagenesis of *FAD2* genes in peanut with CRISPR/Cas9 based gene editing. BMC Biotechnol. 2019;19:24.